Examination of the Back

An Introduction

John K. Paterson, MB, BS, MRCGP

*currently Vice-President and Hon. Secretary of the British
Association of Manipulative Medicine and member of the
Scientific Advisory Committee of the International Federation
of Manual Medicine*

and

Loic Burn, BA, MRCS, LRCP, DPhysMed

*currently President of the British Association of Manipulative
Medicine, Member of the Scientific Section of the
British League against Rheumatism and member of Council
of the Back Pain Association*

T0338504

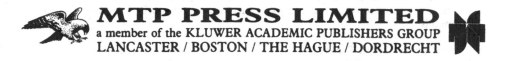

MTP PRESS LIMITED
a member of the KLUWER ACADEMIC PUBLISHERS GROUP
LANCASTER / BOSTON / THE HAGUE / DORDRECHT

Published in the UK and Europe by
MTP Press Limited
Falcon House
Lancaster, England

British Library Cataloguing in Publication Data

Paterson, John K.
   Examination of the back: an introduction.
   1. Back—Diseases—Diagnosis
   2. Physical diagnosis
   I. Title   II. Burn, Loic
   616.7'30754   RD768

   ISBN 0-85200-930-5

Published in the USA by
MTP Press
A division of Kluwer Boston Inc
190 Old Derby Street
Hingham, MA 02043, USA

Library of Congress Cataloging in Publication Data

Paterson, John K., 1921–
   Examination of the back: an introduction.

   Bibliography: p.
   Includes index.
   1. Backache—Diagnosis.   2. Physical diagnosis.
   I. Burn, Loic, 1935–   II. Title.   [DNLM: 1. Backache—
   diagnosis.   2. Pain.   3. Physical Examination—
   methods. WE 755 P296e]
   RD768.P33   1986   617'.56   85-23290

   ISBN 0-85200-930-5

Typeset by Blackpool Typesetting Services Ltd., Blackpool, England
Printed by Dotesios (Printers) Ltd, Bradford-on-Avon, Wiltshire

Contents

Contents

Preface

Low back pain is a major clinical problem, reflected in loss of work on an enormous scale. At the present time in the United Kingdom there are almost 90 000 individuals registered as sick and away from work each day with back problems. This figure has reached its current level following a large increase over the last 6 years and is showing no sign of decreasing. The cost is around £10^9 per annum in lost production, sickness benefits and medical treatment. However, it must be stressed that this represents only about two thirds of pain of overtly vertebral origin, and many other problems caused by spinal dysfunction must be considered.

In view of this and the variety of presentation of vertebrogenic problems, we offer a method of vertebral examination applicable to those conditions clearly musculoskeletal in nature, and also to those conditions simulating syndromes presenting in various fields. For example, cranial pain and a number of symptoms commonly assumed to be of ENT origin (such as tinnitus), and shoulder and brachial pain may have a vertebral origin, as may thoracic and abdomial pain thought to be visceral. Although we do not include detailed examination of the peripheral joints, as this is covered in other publications, nevertheless it must be emphasized that vertebrogenic problems can present identical patterns of pain and that the two may co-exist.

As we are here particularly concerned with pain of spinal origin, we present a résumé of our current understanding of the scientific basis of both pain and tenderness, and their referral. We present and discuss traditional methods of examination and add techniques of local examination designed to identify segmental levels of dysfunction. The latter are derived largely from the work of Professor Robert Maigne. These techniques demand prior discussion of the rationale upon which they are based.

As this book is expressly intended to present and justify clinical examination, we do not include special investigations. While the number of these techniques may at first sight appear excessive and overcomplicated, in that they produce a plethora of information, we seek to simplify the task by offering a simple system of data recording, of considerable value in clinical practice. This is in some instances complemented by an even simpler 'shorthand' method. The therapeutic implications of the findings revealed by this system of examination are reviewed. In addition, we present a series of regional data recording sheets for the comprehensive examination of the spine.

We are most grateful to Professor Maigne for allowing us to make extensive use of his work, in particular his system of local examination. Once again, we owe a great debt of gratitude to Professor B. D. Wyke (formerly Director of the Neurological Unit of the Royal College of Surgeons of England) for further advising us on matters neurophysiological and for permitting us to make use of some of his illustrations. We also have to thank the Editor, *Physiotherapy*, for co-operation in making available Professor Wyke's illustrations. We are much indebted to Mr Malcolm C. T. Morrison (of the Princess Margaret Hospital, Swindon) for the enormous care with which he has made constructive criticism of our text. We wish to thank Mr Zoltan Gabor for the many photographs and Mr Robert Rixon for the complementary line drawings. We also thank Mrs Joanna Vernon for her tireless efforts in producing a legible typescript in record time. Finally, we are most grateful to Mr A. W. F. Lettin for doing us the honour of writing a foreword to this book.

December, 1985   John K. Paterson
                                                       Loic Burn

Foreword

Alan Lettin, BSc, MS, MB, FRCS

*Consultant Orthopaedic Surgeon, St. Bartholomew's Hospital,
and the Royal National Orthopaedic Hospital, London*

With one or two exceptions the pathological cause and the precise origin of pain in the back is unknown. This is in large part due to the fact that the separate anatomical components of the spine and its contents are not individually represented in the brain. At every level of the spine there are, for example, two synovial facet joints which are structurally similar to the peripheral synovial joints. It is quite impossible to say with certainty, however, which one at which level is causing pain if indeed a facet joint is the cause of the pain at all. There is no such problem with pain arising, for example, in a knee joint.

In reality it is possible to recognize certain syndromes or collections of symptoms and signs of musculo-skeletal or neural origin. The recognition of these syndromes is dependent almost entirely on careful and time-consuming history-taking and clinical examination rather than more precise or scientific special investigations.

Drs Paterson and Burn describe in detail the conventional or traditional way in which the spine should be examined and in addition some of the more unconventional tests and physical signs which they have found useful in defining these syndromes, and also their particular method of recording them. It is a sad reflection on undergraduate orthopaedic teaching, or perhaps the time devoted to it, in the average medical curriculum, that such a book should be needed but it undoubtedly is if the enormous social and economic consequences of pain in the back are to be reduced.

Thorough history-taking and clinical examination is the cornerstone of successful treatment, especially so in the management of patients with low back pain.

1
The Basic Neurology of Pain

This presentation is based very largely on a series of lectures given by Professor B. D. Wyke in September 1983 in Zurich. In this, 20 years after the foundation of the specialty of articular neurology, which encompasses the morphology, physiology, pathology and clinical features of joints, he gave a review of its current status.

By the time a patient feels pain, a very complex sequence of events has taken place.

'Information about the presence of injury is transmitted to the central nervous system by peripheral nerves. Certain small-diameter fibres will signal only on injury, while others with lower thresholds increase their discharge frequency if the stimulus received reaches noxious levels.

'Cells of the spinal cord or fifth nucleus which are excited by these injury signals, are also facilitated or inhibited by other peripheral nerve fibres which carry information about innocuous events.

'Descending control systems originating in the brain modulate the excitability of the cells which transmit information about injury. Therefore, the brain receives messages about injury by way of a gate control system which is influenced by: (1) injury signals, (2) other types of afferent impulse, and (3) descending control.'[1]

To quote Wall and Melzack[45], 'current information shows us that the signalling of injury by even the first central cells is dependent not only on the arrival of nociceptive afferent impulses but on the signalling of other peripheral events and on the setting of excitability by central nervous system mechanisms. These contingent controls offer an explanation for the variable response to injury'.

The nerve endings in joints are internationally classified as Types I–IV. Types I, II and III are corpuscular in type – that is they are nerve terminals enclosed in capsules with a variable number of layers. These are the mechanoreceptors, converting mechanical forces applied to the nerve endings into nerve impulses, discharged into the central nervous system. Their response varies with the direction, velocity and amplitude of the forces applied to them, including those forces applied in therapeutic manipulation. Types I and II are embedded in the joint capsules and are, in fact, the only joint capsule mechanoceptors. Type I mechanoceptors are situated principally in the superficial layers, Type II deeper. Neither are present in synovial tissues, there being no nerve endings in these tissues. Type III mechanoceptors are found only in ligaments; they are found in all ligaments, other than the spinal ligaments.

The behaviour of any mechanoceptor, in whatever tissue it may be situated, is related to the thickness of its capsule. This determines the way in which it responds in terms of both time and resilience on movement, active or passive, to traction or to the application of external forces, such as manipulation. Adaptation is defined as the length of time for which a mechanoceptor will continue to discharge nerve impulses, when exposed to a mechanical force of constant intensity. Type I mechanoceptors are slowly adapting, Type II fast. Type I have thin capsules, Type II thicker, the general rule being that the thinner the capsule the more slowly will adaptation take place. A further significant difference between these two nerve endings is the way they behave, either at rest or when moved, actively or passively. Type I receptors fire constantly at rest in the neutral position of a joint at about 15 Hz, whereas Type II do not fire at all at rest. Thus Type I receptors have a static or tonic postural discharge. However, the character of these discharges varies on movement according to the direction, amplitude and velocity of the forces applied to them. Thus Type I receptors have both static and dynamic discharges. Types I and II mechanoceptors have a feature in common, in that they have a low threshold, being very easily stimulated. Thus an applied force of approximately 3 g is sufficient to stimulate a Type I mechanoceptor.

Since the resting neutral tension in the joint capsules is greater than this, there is a static discharge from these particular mechanoceptors. Although Type II receptors also have a low threshold, they have no static discharge; this is because their discharge is velocity dependent. That is to say, in order to recruit them, movements, active or passive, have to be rapid, and this is why they are known as acceleration mechanoceptors.

Type III, the ligament mechanoceptors, have thin capsules – that is to say, they are slow adaptors. But they differ from Types I and II in that they have a high threshold. In order to induce them to discharge, forces of kilograms, not grams, have to be applied, and therefore they have no static discharge. They will only fire at the limits of range of movement, either active or passive, or on powerful traction or on forceful manipulation.

Type IV nerve endings, the nociceptors, are those whose stimulation gives rise to the experience of pain. These are quite different from the mechanoceptors, in that they are non-capsulated. They are subdivided into two types, Type IVa which are plexiform and found in the joint capsules and fat pads, and Type IVb which are free nerve endings found in ligaments and tendons. They are normally quiescent at rest or on movement. They are only fired on mechanical or chemical irritation, the former being very much more common. The chemical substances which can stimulate these nerve endings include irritants such as prostaglandin-E, lactic acid, potassium ions, some polypeptides, 5-hydroxy tryptamine and histamine. These substances appear in conditions of tissue ischaemia and hypoxia, as in muscle fatigue, and also in inflammatory exudates, as in myositis.

The afferent fibres transmitting nerve impulses generated in these various receptors enter the spinal cord via the dorsal roots which divide into two rami, anterior and posterior, proximal to the root ganglion (Figure 1.1). All nociceptive afferents are shunted to the anterior ramus, and all mechanoceptive afferents to the posterior ramus. Nociceptive afferents give off many branches, but all give off one collateral branch which runs to the basal spinal nucleus. It is the axons of these nuclei that transmit nociceptive impulses on, up to the brain, and this is therefore the nociceptive gateway to the brain. For pain to be perceived, this barrier must be traversed. Whether this happens, and to what degree it happens, is dependent *inter alia* upon a peripheral modulating influence provided by the mechanoceptors. This input is derived mostly from muscle spindle, skin and joint mechanoceptors.

All mechanoceptive afferents give off a collateral branch to synapse with the apical nuclei. The axons from the cells in these nuclei then run forward to establish presynaptic relations with the terminals of the nociceptive afferents within the basal spinal nuclei. A crucial factor is that the synaptic transmitter released from these apical spinal neurons onto the nociceptive presynaptic terminals is an endorphin which happens to be an inhibitor. Therefore nociceptive traversal of this barrier is inversely proportional to the incoming volume of mechanoceptive traffic. The greater this volume, the less, if any, pain

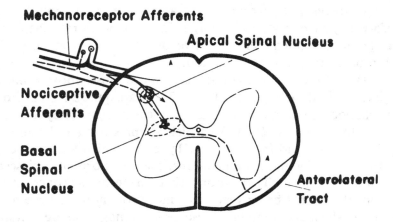

Figure 1.1 Diagram illustrating the principles of intraspinal modulation of nociceptive inputs by mechanoceptor afferents. Description in text. Reproduced from Swerdlow, M. (1981). *The Therapy of Pain*. (Lancaster: MTP Press), by kind permission of Professor B. D. Wyke and the publishers

is experienced. A further remarkable fact is that there is no local enzyme capable of breaking down this endorphin. Therefore, it can only be washed away in the bloodstream, and it so happens that the blood supply in this area is the poorest in the spinal cord.

A number of treatments make use of this system of stimulating mechanoceptor input. The most ancient is massage. A second is the vibrator, the principle being to stimulate rhythmically receptors in tissues from skin to periosteum. Because mechanoceptors have a lower threshold than nociceptors, it is possible (by choosing the appriopriate stimulus intensity) to activate the former and not the latter, the relevant level for most people being between 120 and 140 Hz. Another treatment which involves the same principle is transcutaneous nerve stimulation. In this instance it is the nerve trunks that are stimulated, rather than the receptors, but the principle is the same as with the vibrator: that is to choose a stimulus intensity at which the more sensitive, larger fibres which are the mechanoceptive afferents are stimulated, in preference to the smaller, higher threshold nociceptive fibres. This proves very useful to the physician. Because of the endorphin and blood supply problem mentioned above, 20–30 min of stimulation frequently produces relief from pain for between 4 and 6 h, or sometimes longer.

It seems clear that manipulation operates the same mechanism.

THE CONTROL OF PAIN TRANSMISSION IN THE SPINAL CORD

Nil inhibition

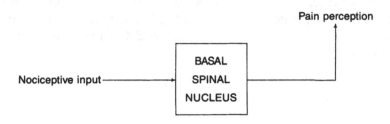

The primary neuron, stimulated by either physical or chemical injury, produces a nociceptive input which, traversing the basal spinal nucleus to the brain, evokes pain.

Peripheral inhibition

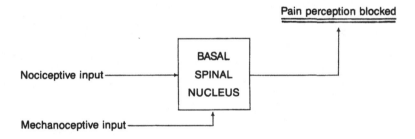

Mechanoceptive input, evoking production of an endorphin in the neighbourhood of the basal spinal nucleus, inhibits pain transmission.

Central modulation

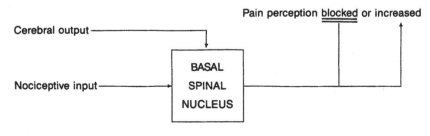

Onward transmission at the basal spinal nuclei may be inhibited by endorphins secreted in the neighbourhood, either as a consequence of mechanoceptive inputs or by central modulation. The effect of such endorphin release, which produces inhibition, is prolonged on account of there being no enzyme capable of destroying it, so that its effect must continue until it has been removed from the site via the bloodstream.

2
The Case Against Individual Muscle Testing

Because of the fundamental importance of the subject, we are fortunate in having had the advice of Professor B. D. Wyke, and his permission to make use of material presented by him in 1983, at the 7th International Congress of the Fédération Internationale de Médecine Manuelle in Zürich.

The relevant experimental work is described as follows. A single articular nerve contributing to the supply of the receptors in a single cervical apophyseal joint capsule is dissected out at various spinal levels. This articular nerve, containing the afferent fibres innervating the mechanoreceptors and nociceptors in the fibrous joint capsule, is then placed on stimulating electrodes, so that the afferent fibres of differing diameters in the nerve may be stimulated at varying stimulus parameters. Simultaneous multichannel electromyography enables one to examine the reflexogenic consequences of this enhanced cervical articular mechanoceptive afferent activity. These reflexogenic effects operate plurisynaptically and plurisegmentally, and in this respect they are identical to the systems operating in peripheral joints.

Figure 2.1 demonstrates the changes in motor unit activity in the homologous pairs of neck muscles on introducing a low intensity stimulus. Since the excitability of nerve fibres is proportional to their diameter, that is to say that the larger fibres have a lower threshold, it follows that, when one applies suitably selected low intensity stimuli to the articular nerve, one may stimulate the mechanoceptive fibres without activating the much finer nociceptive afferents contained in the same nerve. When one increases the stimulus to the nerve trunk to a sufficient degree, one can activate the nociceptive afferents at the same time as one activates the mechanoceptive afferents. The former mimics experimentally what occurs in normal head and neck movements. When one throws in an additional nociceptive input, one

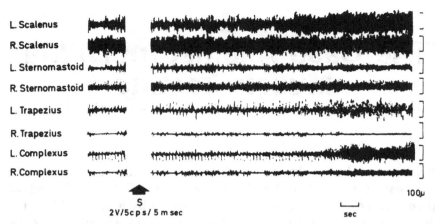

Figure 2.1 Cervical articular mechanoreceptive reflex effects on neck muscles. At the arrow (S), a single cervical articular nerve supplying the left C3–C4 cervical apophyseal joint (isolated by micro-dissection in an anaesthetised cat) was repetitively stimulated electrically for 3 s with stimulus parameters (indicated below signal) that selectively excite the mechanoreceptive afferent fibres in the nerve. The tracings are simultaneous electromyograms from homologous pairs of neck muscles, displaying the co-ordinated, long-duration reflexogenic effects of articular mechanoreceptive afferent activation

reproduces in the laboratory what occurs in a patient who has a painful disorder involving one of his cervical apophyseal joints. The effect of mechanoceptive input is to alter motor unit activity, some muscles showing facilitation, others inhibition, either to varying degrees.

Figure 2.2 shows what happens if one adds nociceptive input by increasing the stimulus to a sufficient degree; the former picture is wholly distorted.

Figure 2.3 shows that the effects of stimulating cervical apophyseal joint capsular nerves are seen not only in the cervical musculature, but also powerfully and reciprocally co-ordinated in the musculature of all four limbs.

Figure 2.4 further shows that cervical nociceptive input, as previously described in relation to the cervical musculature, again completely distorts the previous pattern in all four limbs.

The only project we have come across which endeavours to measure scientifically maximum voluntary strength of the trunk muscles in various populations was carried out by having each subject's pelvis supported while the back was voluntarily extended as forcefully as

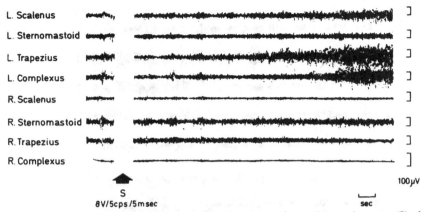

Figure 2.2 Cervical articular nociceptive reflex effects on neck muscles. At the arrow (S), the same cervical articular nerve as in Figure 2.1 was repetitively stimulated electrically for 3 s with stimulus parameters (indicated below signal) that excite the nociceptive (as well as the mechano-receptive) afferent fibres in the nerve. The simultaneous electromyograms (from the same neck muscles as Figure 2.1) display the altered patterns of reflex activity evoked by the additional activity of nociceptive afferents coming from the C3–C4 joint

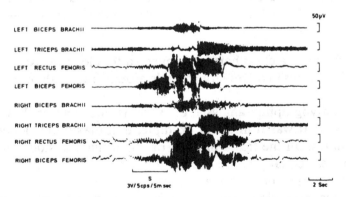

Figure 2.3 Cervical articular mechanoreceptive reflex effects on limb muscles. At the signal (S), a single cervical articular nerve supplying the left C3–C4 cervical apophyseal joint (isolated by microdissection in an anaesthetised cat) was repetitively stimulated for 3 s with stimulus parameters (indicated below signal) that selectively excite the mechanoreceptive afferent fibres in the nerve. The tracings are simultaneous electromyograms from homologous pairs of upper and lower limb muscles, displaying the co-ordinated reflexogenic effects (of varying duration) of articular mechanoreceptive afferent activation, and indicate that such inputs affect limb as well as neck (see Figure 2.2) muscles. Repetition of the experiment with additional nociceptive afferent excitation (as in Figure 2.2) produced a different pattern of reflex effects on the limb muscles (not illustrated here)

9

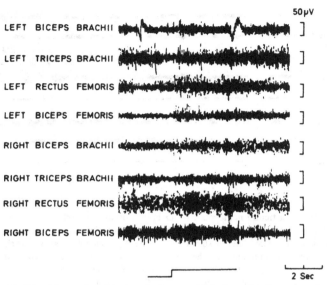

50 µV

LEFT BICEPS BRACHII

LEFT TRICEPS BRACHII

LEFT RECTUS FEMORIS

LEFT BICEPS FEMORIS

RIGHT BICEPS BRACHII

RIGHT TRICEPS BRACHII

RIGHT RECTUS FEMORIS

RIGHT BICEPS FEMORIS

2 Sec

Figure 2.4 Reflex effects of cervical articular manipulation. At the event signal, vertical traction was applied rapidly across the apophyseal joints between the C3 and C4 vertebrae (isolated by surgical microdissection from all tissues other than their nerve and blood supply in an anaesthetised cat). The simultaneous electromyograms from homologous pairs of upper and lower limb muscles display the articular mechanoreceptive reflex effects of such cervical manipulation (the accompanying reflex effects on the neck muscles are not illustrated here)

possible against a chest harness connected to a load measuring force cell[1]. Clearly this involves large muscle groups, rather than individual muscles.

Electromyographic analysis of various movements have been undertaken. It was found, for example, in a maximum sidebending effort almost all the trunk muscles on the ipsilateral side contribute more or less equally to the effort. Thus the value of the so-called quadratus lumborum test seems limited.

'Perhaps the designation of specific function is almost impossible in the back, where we have a complex arrangement of muscle bundles acting on a multitude of equally complex joints. Those who insist on finding prime movers, antagonists and synergists in the genuine musculature of the back will always be disappointed.'[60]

To quote Basmajian and Deluca again, 'In rehabilitation programmes involving muscle reeducation and exercise, it is often necessary to assess the effectiveness of a prescribed therapy programme.

Manual muscle tests are currently the primary procedure for determining muscular strength and progression and regression of strength. Yet these tests are subjective, and their accuracy depends on the training, skill and experience of the clinician performing the examination[75]. In a relatively recent report, Edwards and Hyde[76] stated that there are no *quantitative* methods for measuring muscle function in clinical use today for the diagnosis and management of patients complaining of weakness.

'When a muscle or group of muscles is weakened, there is a tendency for subtle shifts in the pattern of muscle activity to occur to enable the synergistic muscles to generate the required force. This is known as "muscle substitution", and it denies the impaired muscle the intended exercise. Muscle substitution is difficult to detect by current manual testing, which depends greatly on the experience of the clinician'.

In the light of this work, we find it difficult to justify the attempt to assess clinically the strength of individual muscles.

3
Referred Pain, Referred Tenderness and Back Pain Syndromes

As long ago as 1939, Kellgren demonstrated the existence of referred pain following the injection of hypertonic saline solutions into the vertebral connective tissues[2]. In 1951, Frykholm, in his operations on cervical spines under local anaesthesia, found on stimulating the dorsal root that the patient experienced pain in the distribution of the dermatome[3]. If the anterior motor root was stimulated, the patient felt a pain situated in muscles which had been painful and tender before operation. In 1959, Cloward described referral of pain to periscapular areas on injecting for discography under local anaesthesia into the anterior parts of various cervical discs C3/C4, C4/C5, C5/C6 and C6/C7[4]. He identified the painful areas as being C3/C4 for the upper fibres of the trapezius, C4/C5 the upper scapular medial border, C5/C6 medial at the inferior angle. These authors not only demonstrated the existence of referred pain, but fell into the error of assuming that the site of the referred pain gave a clear indication of the site of origin. This has been shown not to be the case – not only by Holt in 1964[5], but also by Klafta and Collis in 1969[6], who performed 549 cervical disc injections over a 10-year period, in an endeavour to evaluate the diagnostic usefulness of pain associated with discography. Pain similar to the presenting symptoms was produced in 22% of cases, dissimilar pain in 67% and no pain at all in 11% of cases. Kirk and Denny-Brown, in 1970[7], and subsequently Denny-Brown et al., in 1973[8], have shown experimentally that an isolated dermatome can vary enormously in extent and, indeed, that the dermatomes should be considered as a neurophysiological entity which can vary almost from moment to moment. Last, in 1978, wrote that 'the dermatome charts of the limb are probably as accurate today as maps of the world were in the 16th Century'[9]. Thus, Mooney and

Robertson (1976), 'It is apparent to us that the localization of pain in the low back, buttock and leg is a non-specific finding'[10]. Discussing the apophyseal joint syndrome, they say, 'on the other hand, the very same referral pattern can no doubt be caused by irritation within the spinal canal'[10]. Bourdillon (1973) wrote that, 'a remarkable property of referred pain is that it can appear to be exactly the same when produced by either two (or more) separate sources'[11]. When one considers the nociceptive innervation of lumbosacral tissues, for example, it is quite clear that any posture maintained over a prolonged period of time can affect muscles, fasciae, ligaments and articular capsules. All these nociceptive systems are capable, severally or together, of stimulating painful paravertebral muscle spasm.

Tenderness is very commonly associated with low back pain and referred pain. 'Referred pain may or may not be accompanied by secondary hyperaesthesiae'[12]. Macnab, in 1977, found that injection of hypertonic saline into the lumbosacral supraspinous ligament could not only radiate pain down the leg but could also produce tender points in varying sites commonly situated over the sacroiliac joint and in the outer quadrant of the buttock[13].

O'Brien, in 1979, discovered that on palpating the lumbosacral promontory via the abdominal wall he found tenderness in more than three quarters of patients with low back pain. In a controlled group of 50 asymptomatic individuals, only two exhibited tenderness and both of them had experienced back pain in the preceding 3 months[14]. Frykholm[3] and Cloward[4] both demonstrated referred tenderness. Unfortunately, the diagnostic use of this phenomenon is as restricted as that of referred pain. 'The certain identification of minor paravertebral muscle strains by palpation is not as easy as might appear, since the phenomenon of referred tenderness can bedevil the most careful examination[15].

The existence of palpable and tender nodules in muscles has long been known. Froriep in 1843, in Weimar, published material relating to them, and they have been a subject of much study in Germany ever since[16]. In Britain they have been frequently described as 'fibrositis', firstly by Gowers in 1904[17]. Another significant paper was published by Copeman and Ackerman in 1947, in which it was proposed that they were due to herniations of lobulated fat[18]. Travell first published a paper in 1942 on the study of these trigger points, in patients with shoulder difficulties, and has published many papers since on this and allied subjects[19]. No one so far has been able to identify these problems histologically. It is therefore reasonable to suggest the term 'fibrositis' should not be used, since its existence has never been proven[20].

'One of the most poorly understood phenomena relating to chronic pain syndromes is the focal hyperirritability of tissues related to painful areas of the body. These areas are generally classed as trigger points and frequently represent areas of referred pain and autonomic nerve dysfunction[21].' With regard to referred pain, while there is frequently a definite association, the site or sites to which pain or tenderness are referred are unpredictable. It is for this reason that referred pain and tenderness may be used only with reservation as diagnostic tools. 'Trigger points associated with myofascial and visceral pain often lie within the areas of referred pain, but many are located at a distance from them[22].' As long ago as 1938, Steindler and Luck studied 451 cases of low back pain with pain referred to the leg on localized palpation in the lumbosacral region[23]. In 228 of them, points were located where needling produced pain felt both locally and referred. Both types of pain were relieved by injection of local anaesthetic in the lumbosacral tender point. It is now generally accepted that the eradication of these points by injection or needling does not indicate that its source has been identified[3]. Nevertheless, such treatments are of considerable help. It has also been shown that injecting saline is about as effective as is injecting local anaesthetic and that simply using a dry needle is only slightly less effective than saline[24]. The possibility of a correlation with acupuncture has been studied, notably by Melzack in 1977, who wrote that, 'a remarkably high degree (71%) of correspondence was found[22]. This close correlation suggests that trigger points and acupuncture points of pain, although discovered independently and named differently, represent the same phenomenon and can be explained in terms of the same underlying neuromechanisms.' Complexities of reference have been highlighted by Simons in 1975, who showed that a lower thoracic point may refer pain to the lower buttock, while an upper lumbar point may refer pain to an area over the upper buttock[24]. In 1976, Maigne demonstrated that upper cervical problems could not only cause frontal headache, but also referred tenderness to eyebrow tissues and that both symptoms and signs could be eradicated by treatment to the upper cervical spine[25]. It is well worth while seeking these points, since they are common, and treatment of them is simple, harmless and frequently of great benefit to the patient.

Therefore, it can be seen that to use the site of pain or tenderness as a means of arriving at a specific diagnosis, indicating a specific tissue, is unrealistic in most of the cases of back pain that we meet. Over the years many syndromes, i.e. collections of symptoms and signs, have been presented as being reliable diagnostic tools. Examples are sudden backache, impacted synovial meniscoid villus, the cocktail party syndrome, the locking of an arthrotic facet joint, the adolescent acute back and slow onset backache and sciatica, or the equinox syndrome. In view of the material presented, such syndromes must be regarded with very considerable doubt. Indeed, in this area it is doctors themselves who have, sadly, greatly contributed to the confusion which is so marked a feature of this field. 'The range of labels used in connection with back pain is a fair reflection of medical ignorance and of factional interests[26].' Moreover, this has had the disadvantage, among others, of persuading the clinician that he has the correct diagnosis of the patient's problems and, therefore, in his persisting in a particular line of treatment, at a time when clinical review would be more appropriate.

4
A Classification of
Low Back Pain

This section is derived from the chapter, 'The Neurology of Low Back Pain', by Professor B. D. Wyke, in the 1980 edition of Professor M. I. V. Jayson's *The Lumbar Spine and Back Pain*, by the kind permission of the author and Pitman Medical Ltd.

Low back pain is defined as pain experienced in the lumbosacral region. The four basic groups are primary backache, secondary backache, referred backache and psychosomatic backache.

PRIMARY BACKACHE

This is defined as low back pain resulting from direct mechanical or chemical irritation of the nociceptive nerve endings embedded in the various lumbosacral tissues.

Cutaneous pain

Intrinsic cutaneous pain presents little diagnostic difficulty and will therefore not be discussed. However, it must be remembered that pain felt in the skin may in fact be referred from deeper tissues.

Pain originating in muscles and fascia

A common cause of back pain is irritation of nociceptors situated in the muscle masses of the lower back, and their fascial sheaths and intramuscular septa, and those in the tendons and aponeuroses that attach them to the vertebral column and pelvis. Such irritation is usually caused by muscle fatigue, mechanical trauma or reflex spasm. Inflammatory causes are much rarer (Figure 4.1).

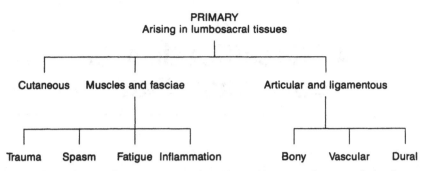

Many different tissues give rise to back pain, with or without muscle spasm (in itself some-times painful). Given this physiological reality, precise diagnosis is generally impossible to validate.

Figure 4.1 A classification of low back pain – primary backache

Trauma

This may lead to tearing of some of the tendinous attachments of muscles to bone or periosteum, or to the rupture of muscle fibres and tearing of their fascial sheaths. The initial pain is due to nociceptive input directly due to the trauma, while prolonged, subsequent pain is due to irritation of the same nerve endings as a result of the chemical changes that occur in the interstitial fluid of the damaged tissues.

Muscle spasm

When excessive motor activity is maintained for prolonged periods in any muscle, pain may develop, and the muscle may also become tender. This occurs because of irritation of unmyelinated nociceptive nerve endings distributed in the adventitial sheaths of the intra-muscular blood vessels, by chemical changes that develop in the inter-stitial fluid of the muscles, in turn resulting from the abnormal metabolic activity of the hyperactive muscle fibres. This may arise from abnormal activity of the receptors located in the joints of the vertebral column (i.e. degenerative disc disease or osteoarthrosis). It may also result from irritative lesions involving segmentally related viscera, especially the genitourinary system. (See section on referred pain.) It will be noted how great is the variety of possible causes and sources of reflex muscle spasm.

Muscle fatigue

Muscles subjected to prolonged work become fatigued and both painful and tender. This is particularly so with regard to the back muscles when they are subjected to postural abnormalities over a period of time, or as a result of the demands of occupation or athletic activity. The cause is not fully understood, but it does depend upon inadequate muscle blood flow and may arise from biochemical changes in the muscles similar to that of reflex muscle spasm. Electromyographic appearances presented by fatigued muscles differ, however, from those in muscles in spasm.[3] It should be noted that backache associated with postural, occupational fatigue is not necessarily exclusively derived from the nociceptor systems in the back muscles, since it may well come from mechanical irritation of nerve endings in the lumbar spinal ligaments or in the capsules of the apophyseal joints or the sacroiliac joints. It is also of clinical interest to note that it can be relieved by measures promoting blood flow and lymphatic drainage, such as massage and heat, and hence is of chemical origin.

Inflammation

Fibrositis has never been histologically demonstrated; therefore, there is no evidence that it exists. Myositis, being a non-suppurative inflammation of muscles, is most commonly seen in clinical practice in association with or as a consequence of viral diseases such as influenza. Pain of viral origin may persist for considerable periods, as in postinfluenzal backache. However, inflammatory causes of back pain are much less common than muscular fatigue, spasm or trauma.

Articular and ligamentous pain

The only common cause of primary back pain, other than myofascial pain, lies in irritation of nociceptive systems distributed in the fibrous capsules of the lumbar apophyseal and sacroiliac joints and throughout the ligaments related to the vertebral column.

Articular pain

Abnormal mechanical stresses can arise from poor posture, from the development of weakness or atrophy of back muscles as a result of ageing, or the reduction of vertical height of the lumbar spine (for example in osteoporosis, vertebral body collapse, or as a result of intervertebral disc degeneration). Articular pain may also arise following manipulation under general anaesthesia or from putting women into the Trendelenburg position (for example), which may place considerable strains upon lumbar apophyseal joint capsules. Inflammatory changes involving these fibrous capsules are most commonly seronegative and seropositive arthritides. In this latter case, the pain is determined exclusively by the inflammatory involvement of the capsules, since the articular cartilages, intra-articular menisci and synovial tissue contain no nerve endings of any kind. It follows that radiological changes, however marked, have no direct correlation with the severity of the backache, and are often absent when severe pain is present.

Ligamentous pain

Irritation of the receptor systems in ligaments is usually associated with irritation of nerve endings located in the joint capsules. It has been thought that static postural support for the lower spine in the erect, sitting and fully-flexed positions of the body is provided by the passive, elastic tension of the muscles, ligaments and aponeuroses, rather than by muscular activity. All these structures are richly innervated with nociceptive nerve endings, and it is clear that backache arising from postural abnormalities of the vertebral column can be readily provoked, as it can by lifting strains. A substantial proportion of the so-called fatigue backache encountered in everyday life results from this ligamentous source in the first place, which may be reinforced by irritation of nociceptive systems in the back muscles and joint capsules. Disc protrusion can cause direct mechanical irritation of the nerve endings in the posterior longitudinal ligament and in the fibrous and adipose tissue that binds it to the annulus fibrosus.

Bony pain

This may be caused either by irritation of the perivascular system distributed throughout the cancellous bone of the vertebral bodies and arches, and of the sacrum, or by lesions involving the enclosing periosteum. The causes of such problems are trauma to the lower back, especially in the case of crush fractures of the lumbar vertebral bodies, the collapse of vertebral bodies as a result of osteomalacia or osteoporosis, or secondary neoplasm, derived in particular from the prostate, uterus, breast, colon, bladder and thyroid. Rarely this may result from primary carcinoma or myeloma.

Vascular pain

This is more common than is frequently supposed, arising from mechanical irritation of the nerve endings in the walls of the vertebral venous plexus, as a result of excessive distension of these vessels by the development of abnormally high venous pressures. The vertebral venous system is in direct communication with veins in the chest, abdomen and pelvis, and therefore elevation of pressure in these cavities is transmitted freely to, and provokes distension of, the vertebral veins. Such elevation of venous pressure may be high in acts of lifting or supporting heavy weights, as the abdominal and thoracic muscles then contract after deep inspiration against a closed glottis. The same mechanism is at play in sneezing, coughing and vomiting, and also in the third trimester of pregnancy.

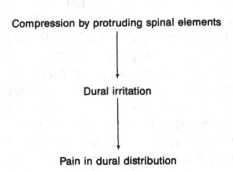

Compression by protruding spinal elements

Dural irritation

Pain in dural distribution

N.B. Compression of a nerve trunk *never* produces pain in the peripheral distribution of the branches of that nerve trunk. The pain produced is derived from the nociceptors within the dura.

Figure 4.2 Effects of dural involvement

Dural pain

While the dural tube has no nociceptive innervation on its posterior surface, it is densely supplied on its anterior surface and in the dural sleeves extending into the intervertebral foramina. Pressure from a bulging or prolapsed intervertebral disc onto these structures produces pain. This may be compounded by the pressure of osteophytes, in spinal stenosis and in spondylolisthesis.

SECONDARY BACKACHE

This may be defined as pain experienced in the lumbosacral region as a result of disturbance of function of the afferent nerve fibres linking the peripheral receptor systems in the vertebral and paravertebral tissues with the spinal cord (Figure 4.3). In this case, the pathological changes are not to be found in the lumbosacral tissues in which the pain is perceived, but somewhere along the course of the afferent nerve fibres that innervate those tissues. Should compressive lesions occur, of which the most obvious example is a posterlateral herniation of the nucleus pulposus of a lumbar intervertebral disc, and if it proves to be progressive, a specific sequence of events in the nerve fibres contained in the lumbosacral nerve roots takes place, which is reflected in the changing phenomena that are presented clinically as the lesion develops.

Because of the correlation between the diameter of nerve fibres and their metabolic activity, conduction in the larger mechanoceptive fibres in the spinal nerves is interfered with earlier and more severely by any disturbance of the blood supply than is that in the smaller nociceptive afferent fibres in the same nerves (Figure 4.4). There is a consequent selective loss of the inhibitory effect of the former on the central, centripetal trans-synaptic propagation of activity in the latter system. If such a protrusion develops further, it may not only interrupt mechanoceptive afferent activity, but it may also irritate nociceptive afferent fibres contained in the sinuvertebral nerve, giving rise to pain in the lower back, in the absence of sciatica (Figure 4.5). If the protrusion increases more in size, it begins to impinge upon the related dorsal roots and their containing dural sleeves, as a result of which the backache becomes more severe and more widely distributed, being supplemented by concomitant, painful reflex muscle spasm. To this may be added the sensory changes of paraesthesia and numbness.

Thus the initial change is increase in pain sensitivity (especially in response to static and dynamic mechanical forces) of the articular, ligamentous and muscular tissues of the back, as afferent conduction normally derived therefrom is progressively interfered with. As nerve root compression increases, this is followed by intermittent or continuous irritation of the smaller diameter nociceptive afferent fibres in

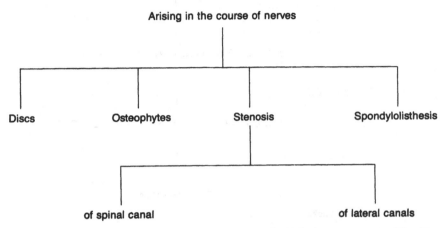

These are all compressive, space-occupying lesions of which the causes may differ. The prolapsed intervertebral disc has been most frequently diagnosed. However, it has been shown that the proportion of back pain due to this cause is less than 5%.

Figure 4.3 A classification of low back pain – secondary backache

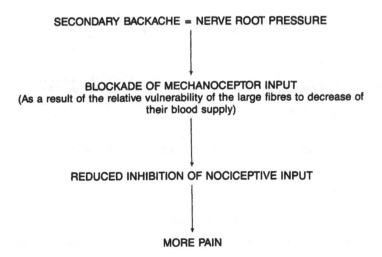

Figure 4.4   Secondary backache – Stage 1

the same nerve roots and their dural sleeves, so that the backache becomes more severe and is less readily relieved by changes in posture or by activity. Compression of the intraspinal nerve roots may persist to the extent that the resulting chronic ischaemia produces degener-

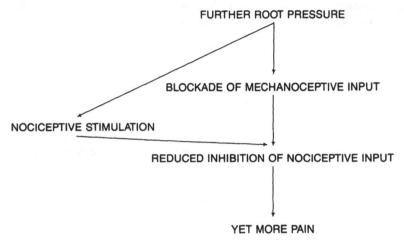

Figure 4.5 Secondary backache – Stage 2

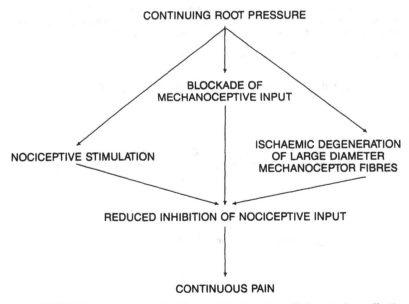

N.B. At this stage mechanical forms of treatment are likely to be less effective.

Figure 4.6 Secondary backache – Stage 3

ation of the mechanoceptive but not the nociceptive afferent fibres carried therein (Figure 4.6). The backache becomes almost continuous, and its relief by mechanical means becomes increasingly ineffectual.

REFERRED BACKACHE

Pain may be experienced in the lower back, although the causative disorder lies neither in the tissues in which the pain is felt nor along the course of the afferent fibres that innervate these tissues, but instead involves some tissue or organ whose innervation is segmentally related to that of the superficial tissues of the lumbosacral spine; this constitutes referred backache (Figure 4.7). The development of a primary visceral or peritoneal disorder may be accompanied by pain (and often hyperaesthesia) in one or more sectors of the skin in the lumbosacral area, in which reflex vasomotor changes may also occur, and this is frequently associated with reflex spasm of segmentally related portions of the spinal musculature.

Recent research has thrown considerable light on this phenomenon, especially with the demonstration that nociceptive afferents from visceral tissues project onto the same relay cells in the basal spinal nucleus as do the afferents from segmentally related areas of the skin (Figure 4.8). Trivial stimuli applied to these areas may induce these relay cells to fire, should their excitability be sufficiently increased by

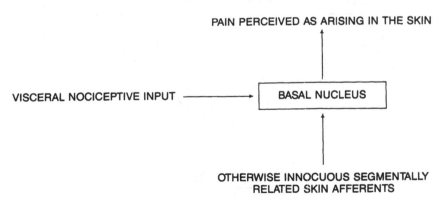

N.B. It is only when a visceral nociceptive input is already in operation that otherwise innocuous stimuli to the skin produce referral of the pain perceived.

Figure 4.7 Referred pain and tenderness

pre-existing afferent activity emanating from visceral nociceptive nerve endings. The resulting pain is then perceived to lie in the skin. Clinically, referred backache is most commonly encountered gynae-cologically in dysmenorrhoea, in lesions of the ovaries or of the Fallopian tubes (such as in salpingitis or ectopic pregnancy) or with uterine prolapse or retroversion and, finally, in carcinoma of the uterine cervix (Figure 4.9). Apart from these, patients with diseases of the urinary tract often experience referred backache, particularly with pyelitis, pyelonephritis and renal calculi. It may also occur in lesions of the renal pelvis, in the presence of an inflamed retrocaecal appendix and in various forms of prostatitis.

PSYCHOSOMATIC BACKACHE

This is a subject in which substantial disparity of professional views has been long displayed. In view of the nature of pain, discussed in Chapter 1, it is clear that all pain is, indeed, psychosomatic, in the sense that it is the individual's personal, emotional response to injury of some description; it is the response to injury that is painful, rather than the injury itself.

Sternbach used the Minnesota Multiphasic Personality Inventory (MMPI), which is the best-established psychological test used to measure personality in the USA, in chronic pain sufferers. This showed

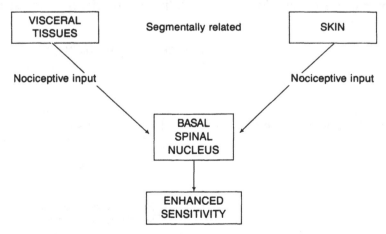

As a result of this enhancement, trivial stimuli to the skin will produce disproportionately severe pain felt in the skin.

Figure 4.8 Viscerosomatic pain

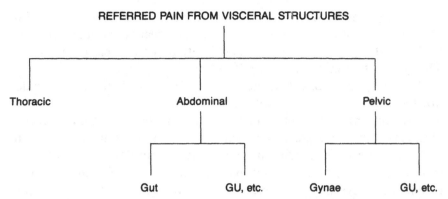

REFERRED PAIN FROM VISCERAL STRUCTURES

Thoracic   Abdominal   Pelvic

Gut   GU, etc.   Gynae   GU, etc.

Even as pain of vertebral origin commonly simulates visceral disease, so also does the reverse take place. (See comment in the section on the relevance of spinal examination to clinical practice.)

Figure 4.9   A classification of back pain – referred pain

that, using measures of hypochondriacal behaviour, there was great similarity between the pattern of the hysterical patient and the back pain patient[77]. That is, that the patient was quite disturbed, and that his attention was devoted to the body. Following treatment, either medical or surgical, the scores tended to drop and the abnormalities decline. The longer the history of pain, the greater the abnormalities detected. This tells us nothing about aetiology but, to quote Woodforde and Merskey[78], 'Psychiatric patients with no physical lesions can have a lot of pain and we can see that personality factors and other aspects of neurotic illness are common in producing pain.'

In an investigation on patients who had definite physical lesions as a cause of their pain, such as post-herpetic neuralgia etc., and in others who had chronic pain but no recognizable physical signs, Merskey found that patients who had demonstrable physical abnormalities scored higher on scales of neuroses than patients who were only neurotic. This indicates that psychological disturbances can be secondary to pain. This was reinforced on going into the psychological background of the people involved, because it was found that those who had purely neurotic problems were more likely to have, for example, disturbed childhoods than those who had psychological problems clearly secondary to their physical troubles[79]. In a profile of the kind of patients he expected to see who had pain and associated psychiatric phenomena, he found that schizophrenia

27

was hardly ever associated. In the severely chronic group patients had hysterical symptoms or personality traits, a great concern about their bodies and a poor response to treatment, psychological or physical. This group tended to do badly if subjected to surgery.

Discussing this work, Merskey writes of patients with pain 'who do not have any recognizable (physical) lesion'.

In the past numerous patients have been dismissed as not exhibiting abnormal physical signs as a direct result of those signs having been unsought due to their being unknown. In manipulative practice, for example, it is common to see patients with headache of vertebral origin who have been labelled neurotic, who do in fact exhibit the palpatory signs of Maigne. It seems to us that a proportion of patients in such studies as we have quoted assumed to have pain of wholly psychological origin might well have exhibited positive physical signs on local examination.

The above material relates to chronic pain sufferers and therefore may not be wholly relevant to the kind of episodic problems commonly met with in general practice. Nevertheless, psychological problems and pain are clearly closely interrelated, and it is often difficult to decide which is primary and which secondary. The latter group is particularly important. Because of this, one should be very reluctant to assume, in a patient who does not respond readily to physical treatment, and who has evidence of psychological abnormalities, that the problem is wholly psychological and not physical. This assumption is commonly made at present.

SUMMARY

It is clear from the above that nociceptive receptor systems are present in many lumbosacral tissues. It is also evident that the causative factors in low back pain are numerous, while the mechanisms of pain production are identical, so that pain may arise from several tissues simultaneously. In addition to this, irritation of any of these systems, alone or in concert, can cause paravertebral muscle spasm which in itself may be painful. It is evident, as has been shown above, that in many instances, in a given episode of back pain, several different tissues may be involved at the same time. It is also clear that the attempt to identify the tissue or tissues from which such pain may be arising is indeed a difficult enterprise.

5
The Relevance of Vertebral Examination to Clinical Practice

THE CERVICAL REGION

Head pain

It is now clear that head pain can arise in a number of cervical structures[2,27–30]. The incidence of these problems is put by some authorities as being one in three. The topography of these conditions is claimed to be 75% supraorbital, 20% occipital, 5% radiating to the ear and up to 5% occiput to vertex, (Arnold's neuralgia)[31]. Therefore, routine analysis of any headache must involve examination of the cervical spine.

Migraine

Frykholm in 1971 wrote, 'In my experience, cervical migraine is the type of headache most frequently seen in general practice and also the type most frequently misinterpreted. It is usually erroneously diagnosed as classical migraine, tension headache, vascular headache, hypertensive encephalopathy or post-traumatic encephalopathy. Such patients have usually received inadequate treatment and have often become neurotic and drug-dependent'[3,32,33].

Pain referred to the head from the cervical spine is frequently both unilateral and recurrent. This explains the frequency of error in diagnosis. True migraine, with its classic prodrome of pallor, fortification spectra, nausea and photophobia, has not a vertebral origin; however, the two may coexist.

ENT symptoms of vertebral origin

It is now clear that a variety of ENT symptoms may be produced in vertebral structures [27,34–37]. Nevertheless, this fact is not widely enough appreciated, and these patients are frequently still regarded with suspicion. In practice, they have almost invariably been given a clean bill of health. Diagnosis is by local examination. However, it is not uncommon for the two causes to coexist.

Post-traumatic headache

There is convincing evidence that there is a causal relationship between past trauma and headache[38,39]. Such cases may be revealed by local vertebral examination. It is clear that anyone with head injury must also have jarred the neck.

Brachial pain

In view of the phenomena of referred pain and referred tenderness, pain felt in the shoulder, elbow or wrist may be vertebral in origin[4,31,38,40]. Therefore, in all cases vertebral examination (and possibly treatment) is relevant.

Thoracic pain

For the same reasons, pain perceived in the suprascapular and inter-scapular regions is commonly radiated from a cervical source. Similarly, pain from the lower cervical spine can be referred anteriorly[31].

THE THORACIC REGION

Chest pain

An example of anterior referral of vertebral pain is that commonly felt in the chest anteriorly, which may simulate visceral dysfunction. Fossgreen, observing admissions to Aarhus Hospital over a period of 2 years of patients suffering chest pain, found that in 20% of cases the cause of the pain was musculoskeletal[41]. Grant and Keegan have described cases where people have chest pain of musculoskeletal origin, this being demonstrated by it being brought on by movements of the thoracic spine, such as twisting, bending or turning over in bed[42]. In such cases vertebral examination is relevant, particularly where routine investigation has failed to demonstrate coronary artery disease. Such examination may well reveal significant abnormal physical signs. Again, visceral and musculoskeletal problems may coexist.

Abdominal pain

A further example of anterior referral is pain felt in the abdomen. This has frequently led to inappropriate surgery (sometimes repeatedly)[43,44]. Vertebral examination may serve to obviate such mishaps.

Back pain

Pain originating in the thoracic region may be felt locally or referred (posteriorly) to the lumbar region and the buttocks. A thoracic source of low back pain is regarded by some authorities as being common[31].

THE LUMBAR REGION

Pain originating in the lumbar spine may be felt locally or referred anteriorly (to groin, testicle or anterior thigh), or posteriorly (to buttock, hip or leg).

It seems strange that, while the medical profession has long accepted sciatica as commonly arising from lumbosacral tissues, anterior radiation of pain from the same tissues is less widely recognized as a valid clinical phenomenon.

6
Traditional Vertebral Examination

The system presented here is widely used, particularly by orthopaedic surgeons and rheumatologists. To this we add a system of data recording for each test, which we hope will be of practical use to the clinician. While each is presented individually, they are, of course, component parts of a comprehensive data recording system, designed not only for clinical utility, but also for computer analysis[53].

In addition, with regard to the global movements of the cervical and lumbar regions, we include a simple, if crude, system of recording degrees of restriction of movement and of pain, described by Professor Maigne[31]. This involves marking the limbs of the 'star' with either dashes for restriction of movement, or crosses for degrees of pain, from 0 to 3 in each case. Where applicable, the two systems are illustrated in parallel.

THE CERVICAL REGION

Posture

There is substantial variation in cervical posture within normal limits, related to individual build and habit, particularly in the lateral view. Kyphosis, scoliosis and differences in shoulder height may be significant, and visible muscle spasm may be present. There may be torticollis.

Instruction to patient

Stand comfortably, looking to the front.

PA view

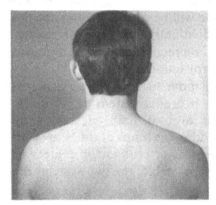 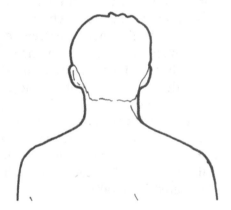

Lateral view

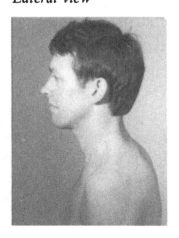 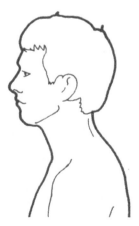

Protracted

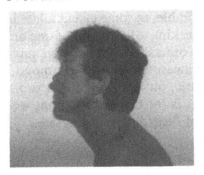 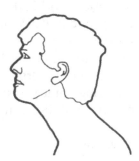

Retracted

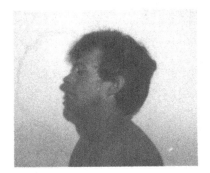 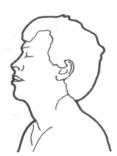

Illustration of data recording

This patient has erect posture in the AP view, but stands with his head protracted in the lateral view. This is unaltered by treatment.

Posture

A P	Before	After
Erect	✓	✓
Sidebent R		
Sidebent L		
Rotated R		
Rotated L		

Lateral	Before	After
Erect		
Extended		
Flexed		
Protracted	✓	✓
Retracted		

Global movements (active)

Variations within the normal are considerable, to some extent related to age and build. What the examiner is seeking is limitation of one or more movements in comparison with the others. Such restriction may be due to pain or lack of mobility. The measurement of these movements remains crude and is not diagnostic, but provides a means of assessing clinical response to therapy. It is for this purpose that we present and illustrate the two systems of recording relevant data.

Extension

Instruction to patient

Look up as far as you can without provoking pain.

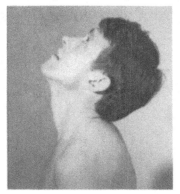
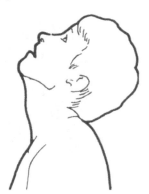

Flexion

Instruction to patient

Look down as far as you can without provoking pain.

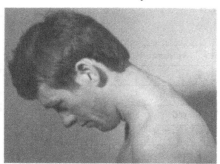
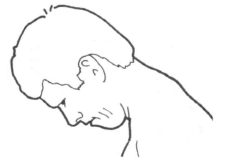

Rotation left

Instruction to patient

Look to your left as far as you can without provoking pain.

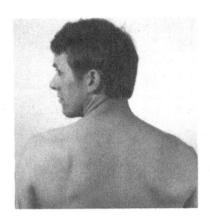 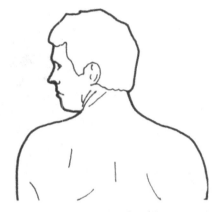

Rotation right

Instruction to patient

Look to your right as far as you can without provoking pain.

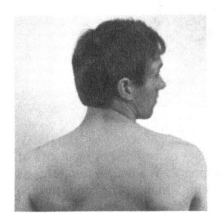 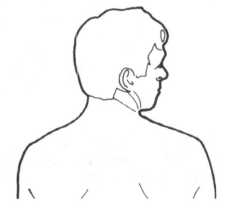

Sidebending left

Instruction to patient

Lean your head to the left as far as you can without provoking pain.

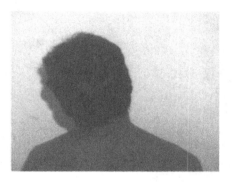

Sidebending right

Instruction to patient

Lean your head to the right as far as you can without provoking pain.

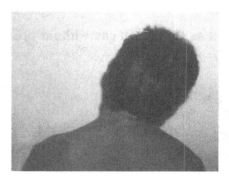

We do not seek to test individual muscles by resisted movements of the head for reasons discussed in Chapter 2. We define the latter as a movement attempted by the patient which is resisted by the examiner.

Illustrations of data recording

This patient has restriction of movement in extension, sidebending to the right and rotation to the left, with moderately severe pain on the movements so restricted. All responded to treatment.

	Before		After		Degree
Extension					Less than 30
	✓				
					30 – 60
			✓		More than 60
Flexion					Less than 30
					30 – 60
	✓		✓		More than 60
	L	R	L	R	
Rotation					Less than 30
	✓				30 – 60
		✓	✓	✓	More than 60
Sidebending					Less than 30
		✓			30 – 60
	✓		✓	✓	More than 60

Tendon reflexes

Asymmetry of tendon reflexes suggests involvement of the nerve roots at the appropriate levels, although this is not necessarily the case[46].

Instruction to patient

Bend your elbow and allow me to take the weight of your forearm.

C5/6 Biceps

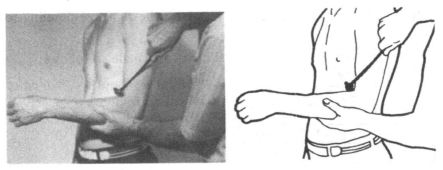

C5/6 Supinator

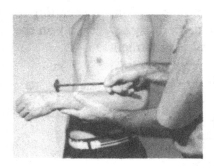 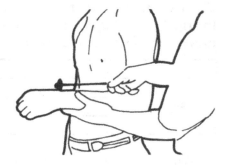

C7 Triceps

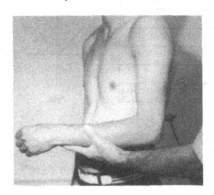 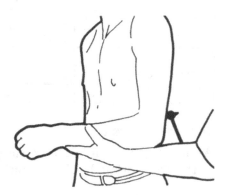

Illustration of data recording

This patient had reduced biceps reflex on the right, responding to treatment.

Tendon Reflexes

Before		After		
L	R	L	R	
	—			Biceps
				Supinator
				Triceps

Entries are made as follows:

Normal response	Nil entry
Increased response	+
Diminished response	−
Nil response	0

Reduced power

The following resisted movements may demonstrate weakness, suggesting nerve root involvement at the levels indicated. Demonstration of such weakness in practice is rare. A common source of confusion lies in the asymmetry of power dependent upon dominance of one side over the other.

C2/3/4

Instruction to patient

Shrug your shoulders hard.

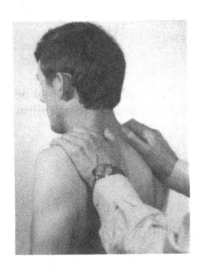 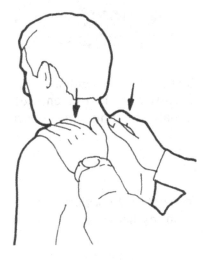

C5

Instruction to patient

Push my hands away sideways.

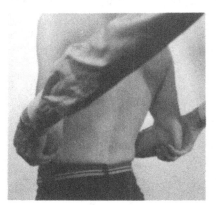 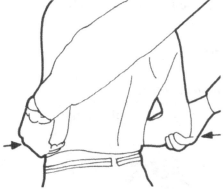

It should be remembered that estimation of muscular power may be distorted by the existence of painful peripheral lesions (e.g. supraspinatus tendinitis or tenosynovitis).

C5/6

Instruction to patient
Push my hands up hard (hands on distal radii).

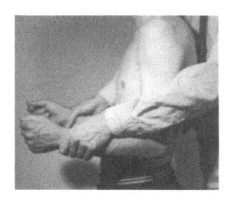 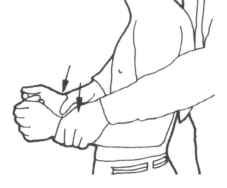

C6

Instruction to patient

Push my hands up hard (hands overlying patient's hands).

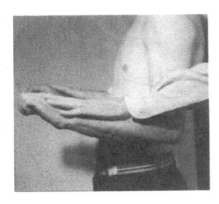 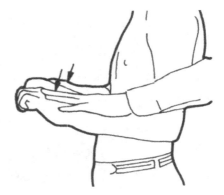

C7

Instruction to patient

Push my hands down hard (hands under ulnae).

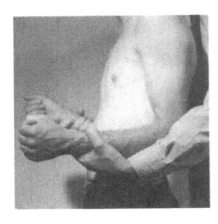 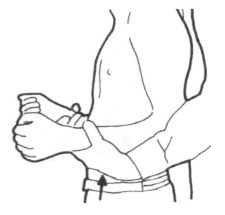

C7

Instruction to patient

Push my hands down hard (hands under patient's hands).

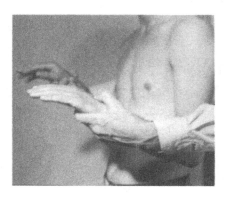 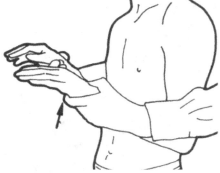

C8

Instruction to patient

Push my thumbs up hard (thumbs on thumbs).

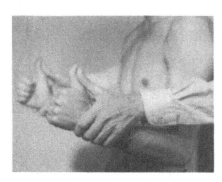 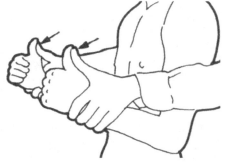

T1 (Also ulnar nerve)

Instruction to patient

Squeeze my fingers hard (forefingers between 4th and 5th fingers).

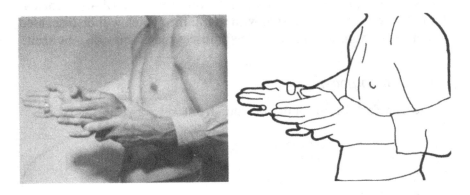

Illustration of data recording

This patient has been found to have weakness on attempted abduction of the left arm, responding to treatment.

Reduced Power

Before		After	
L	R	L	R
5			

If more than one root is involved, further entries require to be made.

THE THORACIC REGION

Posture

General considerations are as in the cervical region. A kyphus, kyphosis and scoliosis may be observed, as may differences in rib-cage formation. These may be associated with sacral tilt, which will be discussed under local examination. Localized muscle spasm may also be seen.

Instruction to patient

Stand comfortably, looking to your front.

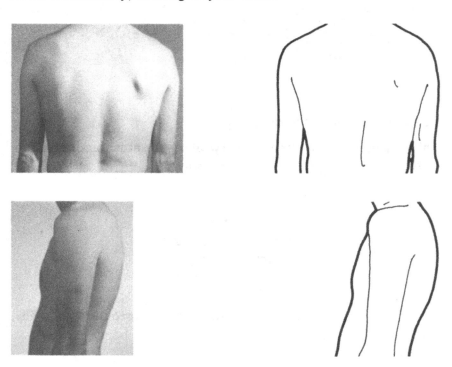

Global movements

Since thoracolumbar movements are considered jointly, we will discuss and illustrate these in the section on the lumbar spine.

Reduced power

There is no orthodox test for muscle power in this region.

Tendon reflexes

There is no orthodox test for tendon reflexes in this region.

THE LUMBAR REGION

Posture

General considerations have been discussed already. Excessive lordosis, loss of lordosis, kyphosis and scoliosis may be observed, and visible localized muscle spasm may be present. Pelvic tilt must be assessed, and this will be described and illustrated in the section on local examination, where its relevance to the spine will be considered.

Instruction to patient

Stand comfortably, looking to your front, with your feet together.

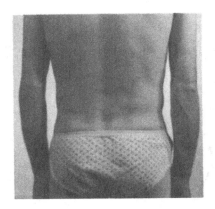
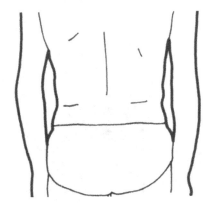

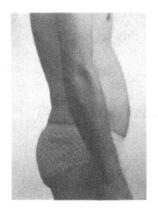 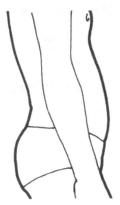

Global movements

For practical purposes, the thoracic and lumbar movements are considered together. Again, what the examiner is seeking is restriction of one or more movements in relation to the others. Such restriction may be due to pain or lack of mobility. It is important to appreciate that the measurement of these movements is not diagnostic, but provides only a clinical means of assessing response to treatment.

Instruction to patient

Bend forwards as far as you can, without provoking pain.

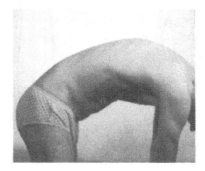 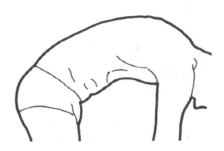

Instruction to patient

Bend backwards as far as you can, without provoking pain.

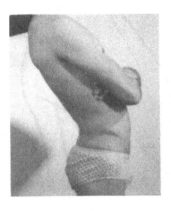
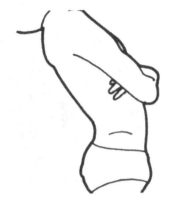

Instruction to patient

Lean to your left as far as you can, without provoking pain.

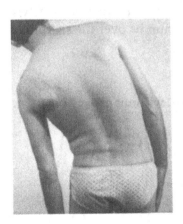
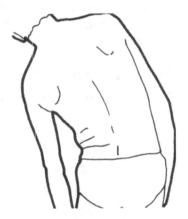

Instruction to patient

Lean to your right as far as you can, without provoking pain.

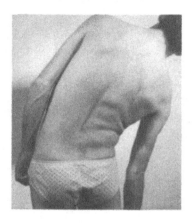 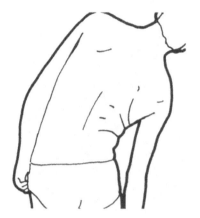

It is not uncommon to observe a part of the spine which remains virtually straight on sidebending in one direction or the other.

Instruction to examiner

Kneel behind the patient and attempt to anchor the patient's pelvis with your hands on both iliac crests, your thumbs over the sacroiliac joints.

Instruction to patient

Twist your trunk to the left as far as you can, without provoking pain.

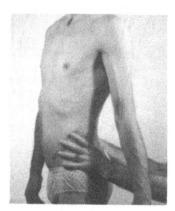 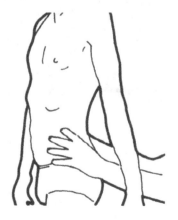

Instruction to patient

Twist your trunk to the right as far as you can, without provoking pain.

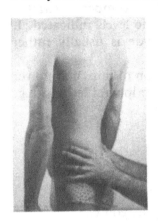 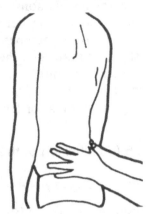

Illustration of data recording

This patient had gross painful restriction of flexion and of sidebending to the right and rotation to the left, all responding to treatment.

Global Movements

	Before		After		Degree
Extension					Less than 30
	✓		✓		30 – 60
					More than 60
Flexion	✓				Less than 30
					30 – 60
			✓		More than 60
	L	R	L	R	
Rotation	✓				Less than 30
			✓	✓	30 – 60
					More than 60
Sidebending		✓			Less than 30
	✓		✓	✓	30 – 60
					More than 60

Fl
SB — SB
Rot — Rot
Ex

Fl
SB — SB
Rot — Rot
Ex

Reduced power

The following resisted movements (better called attempted movements) may demonstrate weakness on one side as compared with the other, suggesting nerve root involvement at the levels indicated. It should be remembered that the dominant side is usually rather stronger than the other.

Again, it must be remembered that estimation of muscular power may be distorted by the existence of painful peripheral lesions (e.g. hip, abdominal or leg problems).

L5 (dorsiflexion of the foot)

Instruction to patient

Pull my hands up towards your nose, as hard as you can.

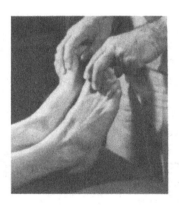 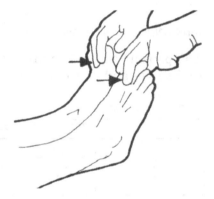

L5/S1 (eversion of foot)

Instruction to patient
Push both my hands away sideways, as hard as you can.

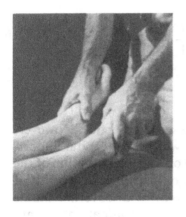 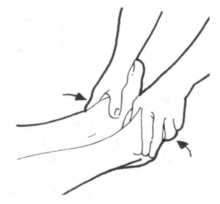

S1 (plantar flexion of foot)

Instruction to patient

Push both my hands down, as hard as you can.

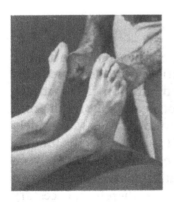 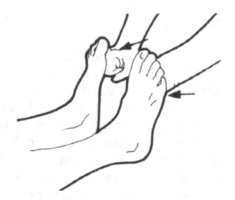

Illustration of data recording

This patient exhibits relative weakness of eversion and plantar flexion on the left, responding to treatment.

Before		After		
L	R	L	R	
5				Lumbar
1				Sacral

Sensory loss

The search for alterations in sensation is common practice. However, with the exception of saddle anaesthesia, which is of capital import- ance, and which is dealt with in the section on local examination of the pelvis, we find such changes of interest only, although worthy of reassessment following therapy. In the event of discovering saddle anaesthesia, either from the history or from examination, instant orthopaedic referral is imperative. It must be said, however, that Mooney regards sensory loss and specific motor weakness as the only true localizing physical signs of nerve root involvement[46].

Reflexes

In 1977, Mooney found that, on injecting hypertonic saline into lumbar apophyseal joints, in 15% of cases tendon reflexes were depressed, this finding being reversed by subsequent steroid injection[46]. This means that depression of tendon reflexes does not necessarily result from nerve root compression. Nonetheless, the following tests are widely employed, and they are commonly believed to signify specific lesions. The degree of resultant muscular contraction varies widely between patients, and unilateral absence or marked difference between the two sides may be a residual result of prior injury. It is, therefore, necessary to interpret these tests in conjunction with other findings.

N.B. Reflex contraction of muscle is generally taken to demonstrate a normal pathway, but see comment above. Absence of one or other reflex or considerable disparity is significant.

L3/L4 (knee reflex)

Instruction to patient

Lie on your back, with your legs straight, and allow me to do the moving.

Instruction to examiner

Raise each knee in turn with one hand, and strike the ligamentum patellae with the patella hammer.

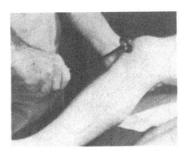 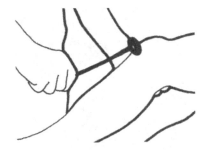

S1 (ankle reflex)

Instruction to patient

Lie on your back with your legs straight.

Instruction to examiner

With one hand, dorsiflex each foot in turn, taking up the slack and striking your fingers with the patella hammer. (This is a more delicate test than by use of the patella hammer applied to the Achilles tendon.) Reflex contraction of the gastrocnemius and soleus (and possibly the hamstrings) may ensue.

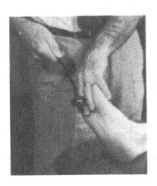 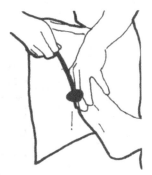

S2/S3 (plantar reflex)

Instruction to examiner

With a firm stroke, run the reverse end of the patella hammer along the outer side of each foot in turn, from heel to ball of the foot. If the response is absent, a root lesion is indicated. If it is extensor, an upper motor neuron lesion is indicated.

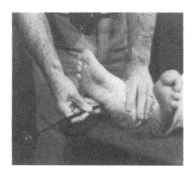 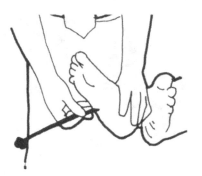

Illustration of data recording

This patient has a nil ankle reflex on the right.

Entries are made as follows:

Normal response	Nil entry
Increased response	+
Diminished response	−
Nil response	0

Tendon Reflexes

Before		After		
L	R	L	R	
				Knee
	O		*O*	Ankle
				Plantar

Straight leg raising

There are considerable reservations to be expressed with regard to this test. First, many structures are involved, and further, either spasm of hamstrings or hip pathology will restrict movement. It is normal for people to vary between 70° and 120°; there is commonly a 10% variation of normal between left and right legs in the same individual, and further many people develop pain spontaneously at no more than 60°. Finally, not only can impaired straight leg raising in some cases be restored to normal by treatment of apophyseal joints, but King has demonstrated that this is also the case on treating trigger spots in the paravertebral musculature[47]. Pain felt in the leg and not in the back may be derived from the hamstrings.

The principal value of this test, therefore, remains as a measure of therapeutic progress, rather than as a diagnostic index.

Instruction to patient

Lie on your back with your legs straight, and let me lift your legs without trying to help.

Instruction to examiner

With one hand on the lower quadriceps, raise each leg in turn with the other hand under the Achilles tendon. Move the legs slowly and note the approximate angle at which the patient complains of exacerbation of his pain.

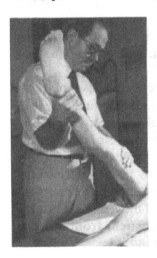 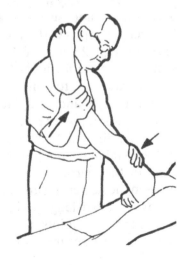

Illustration of data recording

This is a patient in whom straight leg raising is as shown.

Straight Leg Raising

Before		After		Degree
L	R	L	R	
				Less than 30
✓		✓		30 – 60
				60 – 90
	✓		✓	More than 90

THE PELVIS

Very little is known about the pelvis – far less than is known about the spine, because surgical information concerning the latter is available whereas intervention with regard to the bony pelvis is extremely rare. Physiologically, however, the pelvis is perfectly capable of mediating pain, and there is no reason to suppose it is unique in not doing so.

Examination presents difficulties because the sacroiliac joint surfaces are grossly irregular and so formed that there are at least two and often three surfaces angulated to one another. Differences between the joints in the same individual are common. Solonen found variations in 25 out of 30 specimens. In only five were the two sacroiliac joints identical[48].

It is important to remember that the movements of these joints are complex, slight and take place at such depth from the surface that their clinical estimation by palpation is not only wholly subjective, but also must be of limited diagnostic value. In this context, it is of interest that in 1969 Maigne, Gourjon et al. demonstrated[49] the very limited movement of the sacroiliac joints in fresh cadavers by inserting Kirschner wires in the posterior superior iliac spines and levering the sacrum with a crowbar 1 m in length. This produced a range of movement measured at 1 m from the joints of less than 5 cm. It is apparent from this that the range of movement of these joints is small indeed.

Some clinicians claim that they can not only detect sacroiliac movements, but also assess their direction and the supposed resultant adjustment of pelvic alignment. The evidence in support of these claims appears to us to be inadequate and, in view of the above, we offer only one rather crude test, aimed at compairing mobility on the two sides. It must be stressed that this test is subjective and of value only in monitoring therapeutic response.

Any movement taking place at the sacroiliac joint must involve movement of the symphysis pubis and, therefore, examination of the latter is an integral part of pelvic examination. Further, because symptoms arising in the hip or lumbar spine can simulate those arising from the pelvis, examination of the hip and the lumbar spine is mandatory when considering the pelvis. The pelvic viscera must not be ignored.

Some traditional pelvic tests are, indeed, local and will, therefore, be considered under that heading in this book. We, therefore, here illustrate only the so-called ligamentous tests.

Pelvic ligament tests

These are commonly employed and are widely believed to indicate stressing of individual ligaments, as will be described. However, the number of structures involved in these movements is such as to render specificity open to question. In each case, take up the slack and then stress the ligaments by thrusting the limb a little further, to elicit pain.

Iliolumbar ligament

Instruction to patient

Lie on your back and let me lift your legs without trying to help.

Instruction to examiner

Take each leg in turn, flexing knee and hip to 90°, then carry the knee across the midline to the limit of comfort. Gently push the limb further to elicit pain.

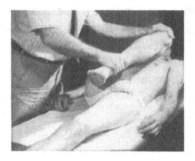 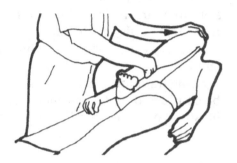

Sacroiliac ligament

Instruction to patient

Lie on your back and let me lift your legs without trying to help.

Instruction to examiner

Take each leg in turn, flexing the knee to the limit of comfort, then carry the knee towards the contralateral shoulder to the limit of comfort. Gently push further to elicit pain.

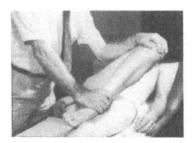 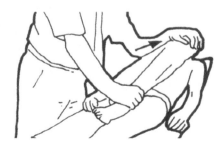

Sacrotuberous ligament

Instruction to patient

Lie on your back and let me lift your legs without trying to help.

Instruction to examiner

Take each leg in turn, flexing the knee to the limit of comfort, then flex the hip by carrying the knee to the ipsilateral shoulder to the limit of comfort. Gently push to elicit pain.

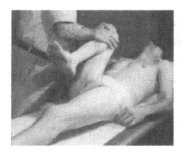 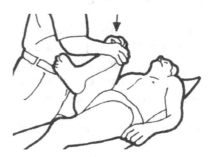

Illustration of data recording

This is a patient in whom pain is elicited on stressing the left iliolumbar and the left sacroiliac ligaments, responding to treatment.

Iliolumbar Ligament

Before		After	
L	R	L	R
✓			

Sacroiliac Ligament

Before		After	
L	R	L	R
✓			

Sacrotuberous Ligament

Before		After	
L	R	L	R

These three tests are the only traditional ones which are not local in nature.

NON-CLINICAL INVESTIGATIONS

The omission from consideration of radiological, ultrasonic, electrical and other investigations is deliberate, as this is a text confined to clinical examination. It is worth adding that such investigations are only needed in a small percentage of cases, where the history and physical signs suggest some cause other than a mechanical or 'arthritic' lesion.

SURGICAL REFERRAL

In general, surgical referral is required when the symptoms and disability that the patient suffers are serious, prolonged or recurrent and do not respond to conservative treatment. Deterioration of symptoms despite treatment is another indication, particularly if neurological signs worsen.

The indications for referral are as follows.

(1) Cervical spine
  (a) instability of the craniovertebral joint,
  (b) persistent symptoms of vascular insufficiency particularly drop attacks, vertigo, tinnitus, etc.,
  (c) intractable unilateral neck and arm pain (especially in the presence of neurological signs),
  (d) evidence of cervical myelopathy,
  (e) bilateral root pain and neurological deficit in the upper limbs.

(2) Thoracic spine
  (a) thoracic myelopathy,
  (b) instability of a thoracic segment which does not respond to treatment.

(3) Lumbar spine
  (a) symptoms of saddle anaesthesia or sphincter disturbance are an indication for instant referral,
  (b) failure of other methods of treatment to relieve severe pain with or without neurological signs in one or both limbs,

(c) increase in neurological involvement, despite other treatments,

(d) intermittent claudication, associated with low back pain,

(e) segmental instability other methods have not corrected.

It is noteworthy that there are two types of surgery: first, to fuse painful or unstable segments, and, second, to decompress nerve roots (Morrison, M. C. T. (1985). Personal communication).

RHEUMATOLOGICAL REFERRAL

If inflammatory arthritides, such as rheumatoid arthritis, Reiter's disease, psoriatic or colitic arthropathy or ankylosing spondylitis are suspected, these should be referred to a consultant rheumatologist. Active Sheuermann's disease or possible polymyalgia rheumatica should also be referred. The reasons for referral in these cases are that full investigation requires hospital facilities, which are also needed for adequate follow-up.

7
Local Vertebral Examination

Diagnosis of back pain is notoriously difficult, in view of the complexity of innervation and the fact that neurological activity is not only widespread, but unpredictably so. This, in turn, leads to the vagaries of referred pain and tenderness.

Traditional examination is primarily of value in nerve root problems, but we now know that disc lesions account for no more than 5% of back pain, and we have already discussed the difficulties of interpretation that arise from such examination. The decision as to whether or not to operate is thus far from easy, as is demonstrated by the fact that, of those cases submitted to surgery, only 50% of back pain and 70% of leg pain are relieved by surgery[50]. For this reason Finneson and Cooper evolved a points system for the evaluation of such cases which has proved of value, in that their operative results have improved by the better selection of cases achieved[51].

Local examination may not achieve a better diagnostic result than traditional examination. It pays dividends in the discovery of trigger points, which may themselves be profitably treated. What local examination does achieve is to indicate the level or levels to which local treatments should be directed. We gave numerous examples of this phenomenon in the section on the relevance of vertebral examination to clinical practice. Of these the clearest illustration is, perhaps, the demonstration by Maigne that in low back pain signs may be found both over the buttock and at the thoracolumbar junction[31]. If the latter are not sought and treated, failure of therapy results, as he shows by reporting a number of cases in which surgery to the lumbar spine had failed to eliminate symptoms, which subsequently resolved on treatment of the thoracolumbar junction.

The system we present is derived very largely from that originally described by Maigne[31]. We are grateful to him for having discussed the matter with us, although he differs from us on certain issues. While he lays emphasis on referral of pain and tenderness within the dermatome, sclerotome and myotome of the relevant nerve root, we believe these phenomena to be more widespread.

The principal problem is to select a term that serves as a substitute for a specific diagnosis, since the latter is so often invalid. The one that translates into English most aptly is a 'painful segmental disorder' (PSD). The segment referred to is not a neurological one, but is rather the 'mobile segment' of Junghans[52]. This regards all vertebral and paravertebral structures at each spinal segmental level as being parts of a single functional unit. The 'disorder' is deliberately vague and remains a matter for hypothesis and conjecture. We re-emphasize our diagnostic purpose as being the accurate identification of the appropriate level or levels of disorder.

Many clinicians regard the assessment of mobility as the keystone to local examination. They believe that 'lesions' cause restriction of movement between adjacent vertebrae and that this can be discerned and evaluated in terms of extent and direction by palpation. It will be noted that all the spinal tests we use depend upon eliciting tenderness, save only that in skin drag and in the assessment of guarding in the paravertebral muscle tone test there is an element of the subjective. We are at pains to make this clear because local mobility testing is entirely subjective, and no scientific validation has been offered in support of this hypothesis.

Indeed, Hilton, in postmortem studies of sagittal mobility in 103 cases, showed that range of movement varied widely, irrespective of age or sex, and within the same individual both irregularly and unpredictably[80]. The objection that this might not be the case in the living is countered by the fact that postmortem changes are likely to occur at much the same rate at all spinal levels. Further, Moll and Wright found similar results *in vivo*, not only in flexion and extension, but also in sidebending[81]. Therefore wide variation in mobility must be regarded as normal, and to use the detection of such differences as the basis for a comprehensive system of diagnosis is not legitimate. For this reason we do not include such spinal tests. This matter is discussed further in our companion volume[53].

The examination of individual muscles to assess their strength and length is not part of the routine spinal examination in this country. Nevertheless, it is widely used abroad. One vertebral examination protocol includes tests of 19 separate muscles[82]. Therefore we feel it necessary to consider muscle testing. Two main difficulties present. The clinical estimation of muscle power is entirely subjective, and to test individual muscles is artificial, as all muscles work in concert to varying degrees, exhibiting reciprocal inhibition and facilitation. This is reinforced by the evidence concerning the cervical reflexes on pp. 7-11. It is for this reason we do not employ these tests.

Signs are to be sought segmentally, both anteriorly and posteriorly. The responsible vertebral level is sought by both palpation and by deep pressure techniques.

The tests are described as palpatory and pressure techniques. While both are strictly palpatory, this division is of practical value, in that it distinguishes between the more delicate and superficial tests (which should be applied first, in order to avoid distortion of local findings), and the grosser tests, demanding a measure of force.

There are four palpatory tests.

(1) Skin Drag is defined as the resistance to movement of the examiner's index fingers over the paravertebral skin. Sometimes the patient feels a difference in sensation between the two sides at a particular level. The implication is not known, but the suggestion has been made that this phenomenon may be associated with local alterations in sweat secretion and in subcutaneous tissues[31].

(2) Skin Pinching is defined as a test for tenderness of the skin and subcutaneous tissues. Because of the phenomenon of referred tenderness (Chapter 3), this must be sought widely, both posteriorly and anteriorly. Not infrequently the examiner will observe a difference in thickness of the skin-fold between the two sides at the level at which the patient reports tenderness. This difference may be eliminated on resolution of the tenderness. Like skin drag, there is no current, valid explanation for this phenomenon. A positive finding does not indicate the segmental level of dysfunction.

(3) The Paravertebral Muscle Tone Test seeks to identify segmental levels at which there is a difference in muscle tone between the two sides. A positive finding, while clearly subjective, is well known to clinicians, as in the case of guarding in acute abdominal pathology. This finding is commonly associated with tenderness.

(4) Deep Palpation seeks to elicit tenderness in trigger points or attachments. Since these may be found widely, they must be sought equally widely.

The pressure tests are three in number.

(1) The Segmental Sagittal Pressure test seeks to elicit pain on applying a midline sagittal force at successive segmental levels. It serves to implicate either the vertebra to which it is applied, or the various joints above and below. Since the cervical spinous processes are impalpable (except for C7), this test is inapplicable to the cervical region.

(2) The Lateral Spinous Process Pressure Test is a forced rotation of successive vertebrae, performed by pressing on the lateral aspect of each spinous process alternately to left and to right.

(3) The Zygoapophyseal Tenderness Test seeks to reveal any tenderness there may be of the zygoapophyseal joint capsules and adjacent structures, in an attempt to define the site of origin of the symptoms. The examiner presses firmly over the joints at each segmental level in turn and asks the patient to report tenderness at any site.

CERVICAL REGION

Skin Drag

Instruction to examiner

Stand behind the standing patient. With a light, stroking touch, run your index fingers from below the hairline to the cervicothoracic junction, the fingers moving about 2–3 cm from the midline.

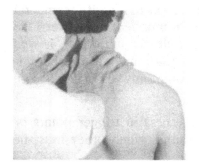
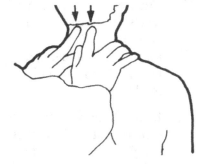

Illustration of data recording

This patient shows a positive sign on the right at the third vertebral level, resolving on treatment.

Skin Drag

Before		After	
L	R	L	R
	3		

Skin Pinching

Posterior Skin Pinching

Instruction to examiner

Adjust the couch to the level of your umbilicus. Stand over the prone patient. Raise a fold of skin between forefingers and thumbs, pinching lightly and rolling the skin-fold in the same distribution as in testing skin drag. Ask the patient to advise you of any difference in discomfort between the two sides at any level.

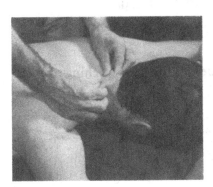 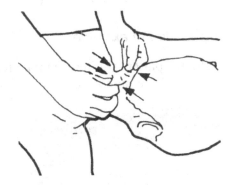

Anterior Skin Pinching (1) (The Eyebrow Test of Maigne)[31]

Instruction to examiner

With the patient supine, compare tenderness on skin pinching of both eyebrows.

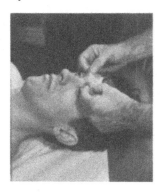 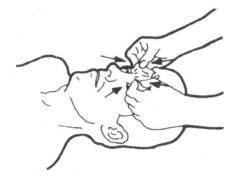

A positive result has been shown to be commonly associated with upper cervical problems[31].

Anterior Skin Pinching (2) (The Jaw Test of Maigne)[31]

Instruction to examiner

With the patient supine, compare tenderness on skin pinching over the angles of the mandibles.

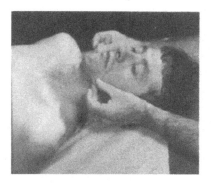 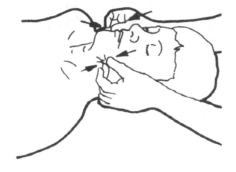

Anterior Skin Pinching (3)[31]

Instruction to examiner

With the patient supine, apply the same procedure to the skin of the anterior aspect of the neck, taking the examination to just below the clavicles.

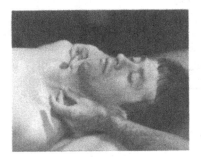
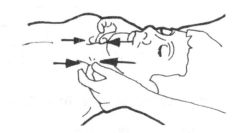

Anterior Skin Pinching (4)[31]

Instruction to examiner

With the patient supine, continue the procedure described down over the anterior aspect of the chest to below the nipple level.

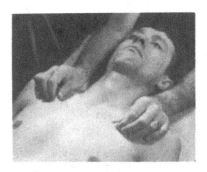
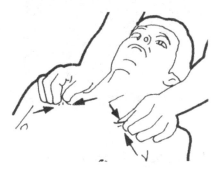

A positive result in all these tests has been shown to be commonly associated with cervical problems[31].

Illustration of data recording

This patient shows a positive sign on the left anterior chest, responding to treatment.

Skin Pinching

Before		After		
L	R	L	R	
				Posterior
				Anterior-Eyebrow
				Jaw
				Neck
✓				Chest

Paravertebral Muscle Tone Test

Instruction to examiner

With the patient supine, palpate the paravertebral muscles transverse to the direction of the fibres, bilaterally at each segmental level in sequence, noting differences at successive levels and between the two sides.

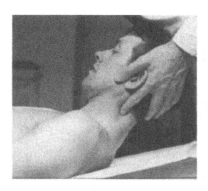 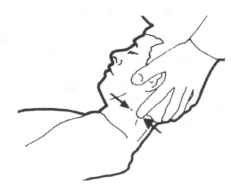

Illustration of data recording

This patient shows increased muscle tone on the right at the fourth vertebral level, responding to treatment.

Muscle Tone

Before		After	
L	R	L	R
	4		

Deep Palpation

This seeks to elicit tenderness in trigger points or attachment tissues. Since these may be found widely, they must be sought equally widely.

No illustration is given, in view of the extent of the examination required.

Pressure Techniques

Segmental Sagittal Pressure

Since the cervical spinous processes are impalpable (except for C7) this test is inapplicable in this region.

Lateral Spinous Process Pressure Test

The last comment applies to this test also.

Zygoapophyseal Tenderness

Instruction to examiner

With the patient supine, press deeply over the posterior aspects of each pair of zygoapophyseal joints in turn. These are to be found approximately one (patient's) finger's breadth lateral to the midline. Ask the patient to report differences in tenderness between the two sides at each level.

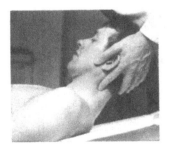
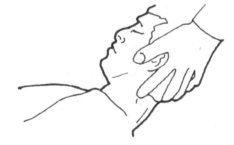

Illustration of data recording

This patient exhibits tenderness over the right fourth zygoapophyseal joint, responding to treatment.

Zygoapophyseal Joint Tenderness

Before		After	
L	R	L	R
	4		

THORACIC REGION

General considerations and comments on these tests are to be found at the beginning of this chapter.

Skin Drag

Instruction to examiner

Stand behind the standing patient. With a light stroking touch, run your index fingers from the cervicothoracic junction to the thoracolumbar junction, the fingers moving about 2–3 cm from the midline.

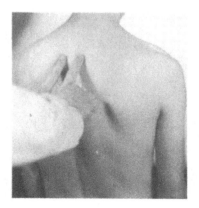 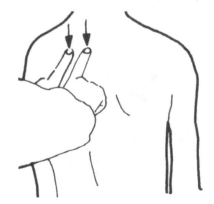

74

Illustration of data recording

This patient shows a positive sign on the right at the third vertebral level, failing to respond to treatment.

Skin Drag

Before		After	
L	R	L	R
	3		3

Skin Pinching (posterior)

Instruction to examiner

With the patient either standing or prone, raise a fold of skin bilaterally between forefingers and thumbs pinching lightly and rolling the skin-fold widely on either side. Ask the patient to advise you of any topographical differences in discomfort.

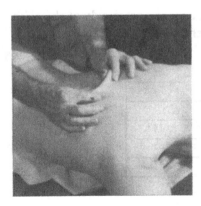 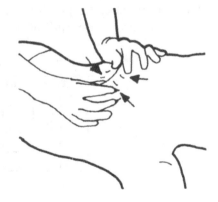

Skin Pinching (anterior)

Instruction to examiner

With the patient standing or supine, seek tenderness in the same way and with a wide distribution.

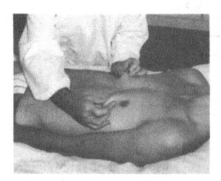 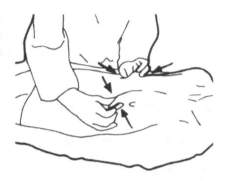

Illustration of data recording

This patient shows a positive sign on the right posteriorly at the fifth segmental level, responding to treatment.

Skin Pinching

Before		After		
L	R	L	R	
	5			Posterior
				Anterior 1
				" 2

Paravertebral Muscle Tone Test

Instruction to examiner

With the patient prone, palpate the paravertebral muscles transverse to the direction to fibres at each segmental level in sequence, noting differences at different levels and between the two sides. Also note local tenderness.

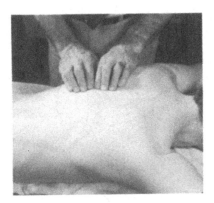 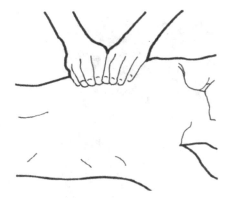

Illustration of data recording

This patient shows increased muscle tone on the right at the fourth segmental level, responding to treatment.

Muscle Tone

Before		After	
L	R	L	R
	4		

Deep Palpation

Instruction to examiner

Palpate widely, seeking tenderness.
No illustration is given, in view of the wideness of the examination required.

Pressure Techniques

Segmental Sagittal Pressure

Instruction to examiner

With the patient prone, press sagittally in the midline at each segmental level in turn, asking the patient to report pain on pressure.

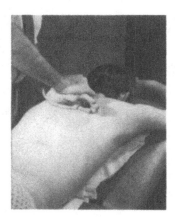
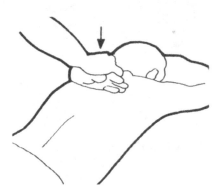

Illustration of data recording

This patient suffers pain on pressure at the fourth segmental level, responding to treatment. The pain is felt centrally.

Segmental Sagittal Pressure

Before		After	
L	R	L	R
4	4		

Lateral Spinous Process Pressure Test

Instruction to examiner

With the patient prone, press firmly and medially on the lateral aspect of each spinous process in turn, in either direction, from C7 to T12.

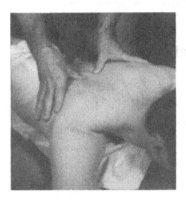
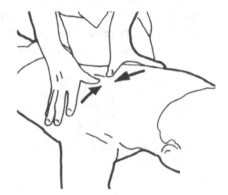

Illustration of data recording

This patient shows a positive sign on the left at the fifth segmental level, responding to treatment.

Lateral Spinous Process Pressure

Before		After	
L	R	L	R
5			

Zygoapophyseal Tenderness

Instruction to examiner

With the patient prone, press deeply over the posterior aspects of each pair of zygoapophyseal joints in turn from C7 to T12. These are to be found approximately one (patient's) finger's breadth lateral to the spinous processes. It must be remembered that in the thoracic spine the spinous processes are oblique, so as to bring each into line with the apophyseal joints one segment caudal to it.

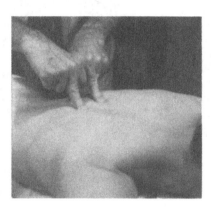 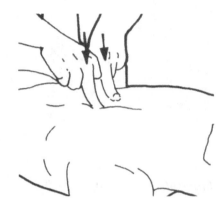

Illustration of data recording

This patient has tenderness on the right over the fifth zygoapophyseal joint, responding to treatment.

Zygoapophyseal Joint Tenderness

Before		After	
L	R	L	R
	5		

LUMBAR REGION

General considerations and comments on these tests are to be found at the beginning of this section.

Skin Drag

Instruction to examiner

Stand behind the standing patient. With a light, stroking touch, run your index fingers from the thoracolumbar junction to the level of the natal cleft, the fingers moving about 2–3 cm from the midline.

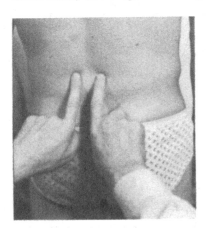 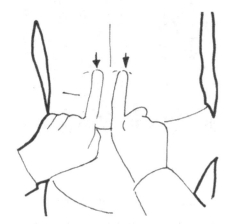

Illustration of data recording

This patient shows a positive sign on the left at the third segmental level, responding to treatment.

Skin Drag

Before		After	
L	R	L	R
3			

Skin Pinching

Posterior

Instruction to examiner

With the patient standing or prone, raise a fold of skin between forefingers and thumbs, pinching lightly and rolling the skin-fold widely
on either side. Ask the patient to advise you of any topographical difference in discomfort. Extend the examination to include the buttocks.

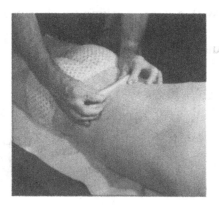
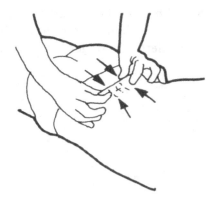

Anterior

Instruction to examiner

With the patient standing or supine, seek tenderness in the same way,
the examination to include the groins and anterior thighs. (See also
section on referred tenderness.)

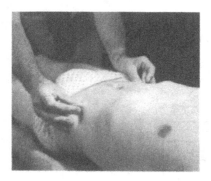
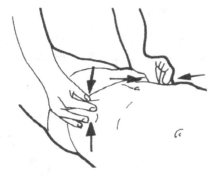

Illustration of data recording

This patient shows a positive sign on the left posteriorly at the third segmental level, responding to treatment.

Skin Pinching

Before		After			
L	R	L	R		
3				Posterior	
				Anterior	1
				"	2

Paravertebral Muscle Tone Test

Instruction to examiner

With the patient prone, palpate the paravertebral muscles transverse to the direction of the fibres at each segmental level in sequence, noting differences at different levels and between the two sides.

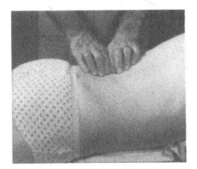 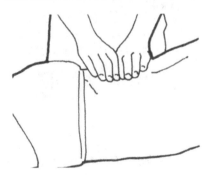

Illustration of data recording

This patient shows persistent increased muscle tone on the left from the second to fourth segmental levels.

Muscle Tone

Before		After	
L	R	L	R
2-4		2-4	

Deep palpation

It must be remembered that trigger points may be found in either or both limbs and particularly in tissue attachments to the iliac crest.

No illustration is given, in view of the extent of the examination required. This must include the iliac crests and the sacroiliac regions.

Pressure techniques

Segmental Sagittal Pressure

Instruction to examiner

With the patient prone, press sagittally in the midline at each segmental level in turn, asking the patient to report pain on pressure.

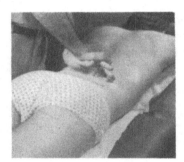 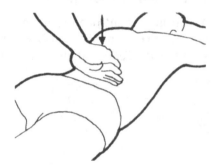

Illustration of data recording

This patient suffers pain on pressure at the third segmental level, responding to treatment.

Segmental Sagittal Pressure

Before	After
3	

Lateral Spinous Process Pressure Test

Instruction to examiner

With the patient prone, press firmly and medially on the lateral aspect of each spinous process in turn, in either direction, from L1 to L5.

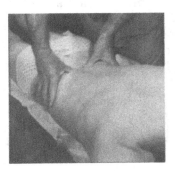 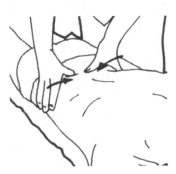

Illustration of data recording

This patient shows a positive sign on the left at the third segmental level, responding to treatment.

Lateral Spinous Process Pressure

Before		After	
L	R	L	R
3			

Zygoapophyseal tenderness

Instruction to examiner

With the patient prone, press deeply over the posterior aspects of each pair of zygoapophyseal joints in turn, from L1 to L5. These are to be found approximately one (patient's) finger's breadth lateral to the spinous processes.

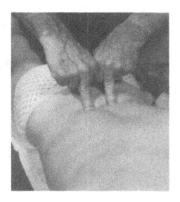 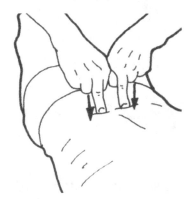

Illustration of data recording

This patient has persistent tenderness on the left over the third joint.

Zygoapophyseal Joint Tenderness

Before		After	
L	R	L	R
3		3	

THE PELVIS

Iliac crest compression

Instruction to examiner

With the patient supine, press medially with one hand on the lateral aspect of each iliac crest. Gently increase the pressure to elicit pain. This test may also be positive in inflammatory conditions involving the sacroiliac joints, and numerous other structures are inevitably involved. Pain may be produced on one side only.

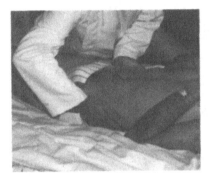 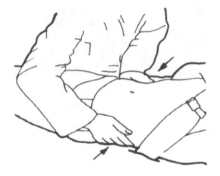

Iliac crest 'separation'

Instruction to examiner

With the patient supine, press down and laterally with one hand on the medial aspect of each anterior superior iliac spine. Gently increase the pressure to elicit pain. This test, like the previous one, may be positive in the presence of inflammatory disease involving the sacro-iliac joints, and again numerous other structures are involved. Pain may be unilateral.

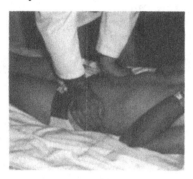 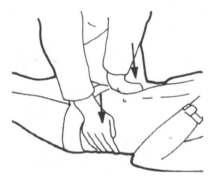

Pubic sagittal pressure

Instruction to examiner

With the patient supine, palpate the pubic symphysis deeply, to elicit local tenderness. Then press more firmly with the heel of the hand to elicit either unilateral or bilateral sacroiliac pain.

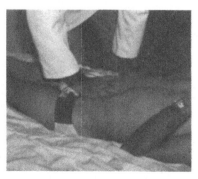 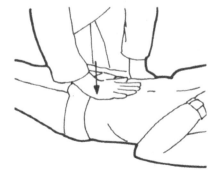

Sacral sagittal pressure

Instruction to examiner

With the patient prone, press down on the sacrum with the heel of one hand to elicit pain. Deep palpation is considered separately under that heading.

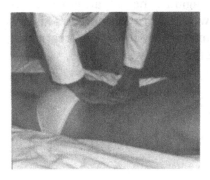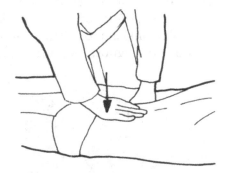

Deep palpation

Instruction to examiner

With the patient prone, palpate widely and firmly over the sacroiliac joints, the upper buttocks and the iliac crests, in order to reveal points of tenderness. No illustration is given, in view of the extent of the examination required.

Sacroiliac movement test

Differences in movement of the sacroiliac joints may be discernible, using a simple test. With the patient prone, the tips of the third and fourth fingers of one hand press firmly down over the sacrum just medial to the posterior superior iliac spine, abutting on its medial aspect. The fingers of the other hand are used to 'rock' the anterior superior iliac spine gently. Movement against the palpating fingers is felt in the majority of cases, and the two sides are compared. This test has value only in monitoring change in mobility following treatment: it is of no diagnostic significance, being wholly subjective.

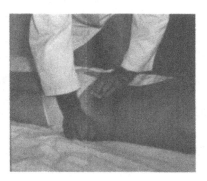 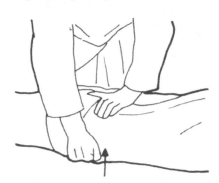

Illustration of data recording

This patient has right sacroiliac pain on iliac crest compression, with tenderness over the right sacroiliac joint and restricted movement on the right, responding to treatment.

Iliac Crest Compression

Before		After	
L	R	L	R
	✓		

Iliac Crest "Separation"

Before		After	
L	R	L	R

Pubic Sagittal Pressure

Before		After	
L	R	L	R

Sacral Sagittal Pressure

Before		After	
L	R	L	R

Deep Palpation

Before		After	
L	R	L	R
	S/1		

Sacroiliac Movement

Before		After	
L	R	L	R
	↓		

SADDLE ANAESTHESIA

We have already mentioned this in the chapter on Traditional Examination. Such is the importance of this finding that we include it in this section under a separate heading. A positive finding makes immediate surgical referral imperative.

Instruction to examiner

Seek sensory loss in the saddle area.

Illustration of data recording

This patient has saddle anaesthesia. Refer for surgery.

Saddle Anaesthesia

| Positive | ✓ | *Refer for surgery* |

APPARENT DIFFERENCE IN LEG LENGTH

The demonstration of apparent alterations in leg length on the employment of a test alternately internally and externally rotating the hip with the knee in flexion, thought by some to indicate a 'lesion' of the sacroiliac joint is of no proven significance; it is commonly positive in both the asymptomatic and in the patient complaining of pain. For this reason we do not use this test.

Further, there is no clear evidence as to the significance of differences in leg length in the aetiology of spinal symptoms. It is, however, in some cases of clinical use, in that 'correction' can, on occasion, relieve symptoms.

Instruction to examiner

Crouch behind the standing patient, his feet together, with your thumbs over the sacroiliac dimples and your forefingers along the crests of the ilia. 'Sighting' along the lines so defined against any horizontal feature at once reveals any tilt of significance. Any doubt may be resolved by 'chocking up' the leg thought to be the shorter on a platform of known thickness and resighting.

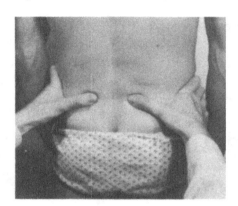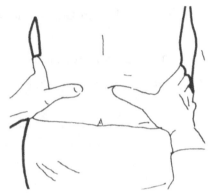

Illustration of data recording

This patient has the right leg 1–2 cm shorter than the left, unchanged after treatment.

Apparent Leg Length Inequality

Before		After		
L	R	L	R	
				Less than 1cm Short
	✓		✓	1 - 2cm Short
				2 - 3cm Short
				More than 3cm Short

OTHER METHODS OF LOCAL EXAMINATION

Musculature

Some authorities, particularly abroad, place great emphasis upon the examination of many individual muscles, and the estimation of their length or weakness. As yet, we have found little scientific backing for this, and therefore we do not include it in this book (see pp. 7–11).

Joint mobility

This is a major diagnostic basis for many clinicians, particularly for osteopaths and chiropractors. We find little scientific evidence in support of this, as we discuss in more detail in our companion volume[53]. For this reason, again, we exclude spinal mobility tests from this book (see p. 66).

8
Regional Data Recording

Data recording in musculoskeletal practice is a matter which has been much neglected in this country in the past. The number of observations to be made in this field necessitates the recording of a substantial mass of data, which can be confusing for physicians attempting recall of information. We have operated a system of data recording for several years, which we have now altered and simplified, in the light of experience. We now offer a series of regional data recording sheets pertaining to the spine and pelvis, to which we have added a history data recording sheet for the sake of completeness. So far as we know, this has not been done hitherto. It will be commonly found that only the history sheet and one examination sheet will be required for an individual patient.

As with the prototype sheets presented in the first edition of our earlier book[53], the utilization of such a form of data recording has the double advantage of providing a check list for the clinician and enabling comparison to be made between data from different observers. The research value of the latter is obvious. The reader may find five data recording sheets somewhat daunting; in practice, separation into the one history sheet and four regional examination sheets simplifies the task of data recording, and the entry of largely ticks or figures renders it both easier and quicker than writing longhand notes. Illustrations are given for each of the tests we describe, and, with a little practice, data extraction from the completed sheets is rapid.

The practical use of this formalized system of data recording is currently taught in our postgraduate courses in Medical Manipulation.

MUSCULOSKELETAL DATA RECORDING SHEET.

HISTORY.

Patient's Name.....................................

Address...

....

Telephone...

Date first seen

Date of Birth

Male ☐   Female ☐

Doctor's Name.....................................

Address...

Telephone...

Serial Number

Dominant Hand L ☐ R ☐

EXAMINATION OF THE BACK

Peculiar Features

HABIT

Work

Heavy	Awkward	Light	Sitting +	S/Emp

Home

Housework+	Shopping+	Gardening+	Under 5's .

Sports

Car

Short	Long	Auto	P/St	0-5000	5-15000	15-25000	More

REGIONAL DATA RECORDING

PREVIOUS RELATED EPISODES

First Attack

Sudden	C	T	L	Bed	Restricted	Off work	Recurring	Worsening	Improving

NON-RELATED HISTORY

Labours		Operations	
Normal			
Abnormal			

Injuries involving fracture

	L	R
Cranial		
Vertebro-pelvic		
Brachial		
Crural		

Soft-tissue injuries

	L	R

MEDICAL CONDITIONS

	Past	Current		Past	Current
Malignant Disease			Osteoarthrosis		
Psoriasis			Osteoporosis		
Gout			Osteomalacia		
Diabetes Mellitus			Osteochondritis		
Rheumatoid Arthritis			Polymyalgia Rheumatica		
Ankylosing Spondylitis			Vascular Disease		
Sero-negative Arthropathy			Anticoagulant Therapy		
Steroid Therapy					

97

PREVIOUS THERAPY	Improved	ISQ	Worse	Doctor	Physio	Osteo	Other
Heat & Exercises							
SWD, U/S or I/F							
Manipulation – Painful							
Manipulation – Painless							
Manipulation under GA							
Collar, Corset etc							
Traction – Sustained							
Traction – Intermittent							
Traction – Continuous							
Injections							
Surgery							
Other							

98

PRESENT EPISODE

Sudden Onset		Unexplained Weight Loss	
Duration – days		Drop Attacks	
Duration – Weeks		Vertigo	
Duration – Months		Saddle Anaesthesia	
Duration – Years		Sphincter Prob;ems	

Precipitating Factors

CURRENT THERAPY

Preparation	Dose	Frequency	Result			Side Effects
			Good	Moderate	Poor	

PAIN

Level	L	M	R	L	M	R	L	M	R	L	M	R
	Initial						After therapy					
Cranial												
Cervical												
Brachial												
Thoracic												
Lumbar												
Sacral												
Crural												

ALTERED SENSATION

Level	Initial						After therapy											
	L	M	R	L	M	R	L	M	R	L	M	R	L	M	R	L	M	R
Cranial																		
Cervical																		
Brachial																		
Thoracic																		
Lumbar																		
Sacral																		
Crural																		

Comment

100

MUSCULOSKELETAL DATA RECORDING SHEET

EXAMINATION – CERVICAL

Patient's name...

Serial No: ☐

Posture

A P	Before	After				
Erect						
Sidebent R						
Sidebent L						
Rotated R						
Rotated L						

Lateral	Before	After				
Erect						
Extended						
Flexed						
Protracted						
Retracted						

101

Global Movements

	Before	After	Degree	L	R	L	R	L	R	L	R
Extension			Less than 30								
			30 – 60								
			More than 60								
Flexion			Less than 30								
			30 – 60								
			More than 60								
	L	R	L	R							
Rotation			Less than 30								
			30 – 60								
			More than 60								
Sidebending			Less than 30								
			30 – 60								
			More than 60								

Tendon Reflexes

	Before		After						
	L	R	L	R	L	R	L	R	L	R
Biceps										
Supinator										
Triceps										

Reduced Power

Before		After						
L	R	L	R	L	R	L	R	L	R

Skin Drag

Before		After											
L	R	L	R	L	R	L	R	L	R	L	R	L	R

Skin Pinching

	Before		After					
	L	R	L	R	L	R	L	R
Posterior								
Anterior-Eyebrow								
Jaw								
Neck								
Chest								

Zygoapophyseal Joint Tenderness

Before		After										
L	R	L	R	L	R	L	R	L	R	L	R

Muscle Tone

Before		After				
L	R	L	R	L	R

Therapy

Initial					
Manipulation					
Injection – various					
Auto-suspension					
Traction					
Drugs – specify					
El.Acupuncture					
TNS					
Other					

Comment

MUSCULOSKELETAL DATA RECORDING SHEET.

EXAMINATION — THORACIC.

Patient's Name...

Serial Number ☐

Posture

AP	Before	After					
Erect							
Sidebent – L							
Sidebent – R							
Rotated – L							
Rotated – R							

Lateral	Before	After			
Erect					
Extended					
Flexed					

105

Skin Drag

Before		After							
L	R	L	R	L	R	L	R	L	R

Skin Pinching

Before		After							
L	R	L	R	L	R	L	R	L	R
Posterior									
Anterior									

Segmental Sagittal Pressure

Before		After							
L	R	L	R	L	R	L	R	L	R

Muscle Tone

Before		After							
L	R	L	R	L	R	L	R	L	R

Lateral Spinous Process Pressure

Before		After							
L	R	L	R	L	R	L	R	L	R

Zygoapophyseal Joint Tenderness

Before		After							
L	R	L	R	L	R	L	R	L	R

Therapy

Initial				
Manipulation				
Injection – Various				
Auto-Suspension				
Traction				
Drugs – Specify				
El.Acupuncture				
TNS				
Other				

Comment

4.

Serial No:

MUSCULOSKELETAL DATA RECORDING SHEET

EXAMINATION - LUMBAR

Patient's name..

Posture

A P	Before	After					
Erect							
Sidebent R							
Sidebent L							
Rotated R							
Rotated L							

Lateral	Before	After					
Erect							
Extended							
Flexed							
Protracted							
Retracted							

Global Movements

	Before	After	Degree	L	R	L	R	L	R	L	R
Extension			Less than 30								
			30 – 60								
			More than 60								
Flexion			Less than 30								
			30 – 60								
			More than 60								
Rotation	L	R	Less than 30								
			30 – 60								
			More than 60								
Sidebending			Less than 30								
			30 – 60								
			More than 60								

Tendon Reflexes

	Before		After									
	L	R	L	R		L	R	L	R	L	R	L	R
Knee												
Ankle												
Plantar												

Reduced Power

Before		After						
L	R	L	R	L	R	L	R	L	R

Straight Leg Raising

	Before		After		Degree					
	L	R	L	R		L	R	L	R	L	R
					Less than 30					
					30 – 60					
					60 – 90					
					More than 90					

Skin Pinching

Before		After					
L	R	L	R	L	R	L	R

		Posterior
		Anterior 1
		" 2

Skin Drag

Before		After					
L	R	L	R	L	R	L	R

Segmental Sagittal Pressure

Before		After					
L	R	L	R	L	R	L	R

Muscle Tone

Before		After					
L	R	L	R	L	R	L	R

Lateral Spinous Process Pressure

Before		After					
L	R	L	R	L	R	L	R

Zygoapophyseal Joint Tenderness

Before		After					
L	R	L	R	L	R	L	R

Therapy

Initial						
Manipulation						
Injection – Various						
Auto-suspension						
Traction						
Drugs – specify						
El.Acupuncture						
TNS						
Other						

Comment

MUSCULOSKELETAL DATA RECORDING SHEET.

EXAMINATION - PELVIC.

Patient's Name..........................

Serial No. [ ]

Iliolumbar Ligament

Before		After							R
L	R	L	R	L	R	L	R	L	

Sacrotuberous Ligament

Before		After							R
L	R	L	R	L	R	L	R	L	

Iliac Crest Compression

Before		After							R
L	R	L	R	L	R	L	R	L	

Pubic Sagittal Pressure

Before		After							R
L	R	L	R	L	R	L	R	L	

Sacroiliac Ligament

Before		After							R
L	R	L	R	L	R	L	R	L	

Iliac Crest "Separation"

Before		After							R
L	R	L	R	L	R	L	R	L	

Sacral Sagittal Pressure

Before		After							R
L	R	L	R	L	R	L	R	L	

Sacroiliac Movement

Before		After												
L	R	L	R	L	R	L	R	L	R	L	R	L	R	

Deep Palpation

Before		After									
L	R	L	R	L	R	L	R	L	R	L	R

Saddle Anaesthesia

Positive	

Apparent Leg Length Inequality

Before		After									
L	R	L	R	L	R	L	R	L	R	L	R

Less than 1cm Short

1 – 2cm Short

2 – 3cm Short

More than 3cm Short

Comment

113

9
Therapeutic Implications

The object of traditional examination techniques is to aid in making a diagnosis. In view of the neurophysiological factors discussed in Chapter 1 and the dual phenomena of referred pain and referred tenderness, it is on this basis alone impossible to substantiate a diagnosis with any real precision, and further information must be sought, as described in Chapter 7. The data so produced will commonly permit the identification of levels of segmental dysfunction, rather than demonstrating the anatomical structure in which the pain originates. The latter is usually impossible, although the site may be reasonably accurately defined.

This being the case, the choice of therapy must depend upon two major factors: first, the likelihood of efficacy of a particular therapy (in the absence of a diagnosis) and second, the absence of contra-indication in respect of the treatment considered. Having defined the elective site of therapy (the segmental level of dysfunction, either on the left or on the right) its application remains largely empirical.

'In a general survey of the treatment of low back pain, it is pertinent to remember that with most of our patients we are uncertain of the true cause of their pain, and that present day methods of treatment suffer from this lack of knowledge'[54]. The fact is that, at present, 'in the great majority of cases we do not know the tissue or tissues from which back pain is originating or the cause of that pain. In the absence of an accurate diagnosis, controlled therapy is not possible. Therapeutic procedures, then, merely become empirical exercises'[55].

Equipped with the limited diagnostic information described, having identified the elective site of therapy, a number of therapies must be considered against an understanding of articular neurophysiology.

DRUGS

Huskisson, in 1974, wrote, 'The clinician choosing a drug for his rheumatic patient is presented with a bewildering array of analgesic, anti-inflammatory, immunosuppressive and other medicines. The same drug also appears under different names, in different dosages, combinations and formulations'[56]. Carson Dick, in 1978, writes of this 'tidal wave of anti-rheumatic drugs' and suggests that clinicians faced with this choice should endeavour to use the minimum number of drugs possible, in order to reduce confusion, and use the minimum amount of any single drug that achieves its therapeutic objectives[57]. Lee *et al.*, in 1974, noted that present day prescribing habits leave much to be desired[58]. With regard to the mode of action of anti-rheumatic drugs, 'no unifying hypothesis currently in existence explains with any conviction why a variety of antirheumatic drugs work and, in particular, there is a dearth of evidence suggesting any degree of specificity[59]. These drugs have widespread biological effects on mediators. 'In fact none of the known biological effects of anti-rheumatic drugs can be produced in support of any existing theory which would explain why these drugs relieve the symptoms of many thousands of patients'[57].

It is of interest that 'the mode of action of antirheumatic drugs is completely unknown, and too often authorities have produced evidence ''validating'' a particular mechanism, rather than attempting to find evidence which is discordant'[57]. The fact that the mode of action of antirheumatic drugs remains 'completely unknown' may surprise many clinicians. In view of this, however, the case for therapeutic empiricism in musculoskeletal disorders is strong.

Nevertheless, these preparations are probably the most frequently deployed 'therapeutic tool' for musculoskeletal conditions, particularly in general practice, where they are prescribed on an enormous scale. In view of the relatively high incidence of undesirable and sometimes dangerous side-effects, while they are frequently helpful in a manner and degree both unpredictable, other treatments must be given careful consideration.

MASSAGE

Although it is of substantial value to the osteopath and physiotherapist, its mode of employment is a positive disadvantage to the medical practitioner in view of its time-consuming nature, in respect of both length and number of sessions which may be required.

TRACTION

Currently traction is out of favour with a large proportion of the medical profession because a number of trials have failed to demonstrate its efficacy. This is hardly surprising, in view of the fact that, for reasons already given, a valid diagnosis is rare. Because traction is generally harmless, it should retain a place as an empirical option. Again, its chief disadvantage lies in its time consuming nature.

COLLARS AND CORSETS

These are commonly prescribed, but their mode of action is unknown. Once more, their use is empirical and, in the case of collars, in certain circumstances can be dangerous. Collars worn by motor car drivers, in the presence of degenerative changes in the cervical spine, can distort proprioception, and fatal accidents have ensued[60]. The use of either is justified so long as the patient benefits (which is by no means always the case). This is why Professor Jayson has said that the ideal corset is one that spontaneously falls apart after 6 months' use, thus compelling the physician to reassess the situation[61].

OTHER PHYSIOTHERAPEUTIC MEASURES

Several other therapies have become established over the years, and are very commonly used, notably in hospital practice. These include heat and cold, shortwave diathermy, ultrasound and interferential therapy. All enjoyed great popularity some years ago, but they have fallen out of favour due to lack of validation as to efficacy. Nevertheless, they are generally harmless and still have a part to play, as they have their successes.

EXERCISE AND EXERCISES

No positive correlation has been demonstrated between physical fitness and the prevention of back pain. Nonetheless, exercise is frequently encouraged, in the belief that it will reduce the risk of musculoskeletal problems, and exercises remain the most frequently prescribed physical remedy in this field worldwide[62]. Recent work has altered attitudes as to which exercises are appropriate. Professor Jayson wrote,

'In my own view, the right sort of exercises for most back pain patients are isometric exercises, aimed at strengthening the paraspinal and abdominal muscles'[61]. Nachemson, over 20 years of measuring intradiscal pressures in the lumbar spine, has shown that some commonly prescribed exercises increase the load on the lumbar spine to such an extent that intradiscal pressures reach levels as high as those measured in standing and leaning forwards with weights in the hands[62]. This rise is particularly marked in sitting-up exercises, with the knees either flexed or extended. Therefore, it must be accepted that these should be avoided, which is one of the reasons why isometric exercises are currently in favour.

POSTURE AND PROPHYLAXIS

Since many musculoskeletal problems appear to be derived from poor posture, either at work or domestically, it is pertinent to consider the prophylactic measures which may counter this. With regard to the cervical spine, let us consider the resting posture. Extension of the neck can pull on cervicobrachial nerve roots[63]. On the other hand, flexion can pull on the cervical roots and sleeves[64], and osteophytic bone can be pressed against the spinal cord[65]. Therefore the best resting posture for the neck must be a neutral position, with support if need be in the evening or possibly the use of a soft collar (in particular in cases with morning pain). With regard to activity, any activity producing pain (if persisted in) should be curtailed. This is particularly relevant with regard to modification of work habit. Thus the typist who develops discomfort or pain as the day wears on should be advised to 'walk it off' the moment discomfort appears. Carrying luggage is also a frequent source of neck pain, and should be avoided if possible; if avoidance is not possible, the load should be evenly divided between the two hands. Driving is particularly hard on necks; collars should never been worn on driving, since they distort cervical proprioceptive reflexes, and road traffic accidents can result from loss of muscular control[66]. On the advent of discomfort or pain, the driver should be encouraged to stop his motor car and to walk about for a few minutes.

With regard to the thoracic spine, the ideal resting posture is lying on the floor, with the knees bent and a pillow under the head. Activities adversely affecting the thoracic spine are those such as hanging out the washing or curtains, pushing motor cars or mowing lawns, and advice with regard to the curtailment of these activities should be given. The ideal angle of the trunk in driving is 120° (according to Andersson in 1974)[67]. It is often worthwhile varying this angle at intervals on a long journey.

With regard to the low back, the fog of war descends. Traditionally, the tendency to make a single diagnosis for all cases of back pain has led to restricted postural advice, stressing either kyphosis[68] or lordosis[69]. However, Nachemson in 1976 wrote, 'we do not know where the pain comes from, or at what level we are treating the patient, i.e. at the level of the motion segment, at the level of the dorsal horn neuron in the spinal cord, or at higher levels in the brain'[70]. All are now agreed that back pain is multifactorial in origin. Thus Weinstein in 1977 showed that both stenosis and lordosis were causes of pain[71]. Hutton and Adams in 1980 were able to show that both flexion and extension can be factors in the causation of pain and of degeneration of the spine[72]. It is noteworthy how recent this work is. Another myth, sadly, is that concerning the value of training in lifting. Wood[73] showed that, between 1961 and 1967, there was an increase in episodes of back pain of 22%, and in duration of attack of 30% – this at a time when training and advice with regard to lifting was widely available. Troup in 1979 came to the conclusion that, 'there is little evidence based on prospective epidemiological studies to prove the value of training, but there is no doubt that a well prepared programme can have satisfactory results, even if one of the mechanisms is the Hawthorn effect'[74]. The latter is the initial and transient improvement which may follow any change in management.

ACUPUNCTURE, ELECTROACUPUNCTURE AND TNS

Regardless of the theoretical claims made in respect of these therapies, in a proportion of cases they afford relief of symptoms. They should not be discarded for want of validation. Indeed, never has acupuncture been so widely used by the medical profession as at present, and it is commonly employed in pain clinics, as it is harmless and frequently of value. We now have a rather better understanding of transcutaneous nerve stimulation (TNS), which works by stimulating nerve trunks as distinct from the receptors, the latter of which is the mechanism operating in massage and manipulation. Its chief advantage lies in its use by the patient with intractable pain (e.g. brachial plexus injuries) who may treat himself as required.

INJECTIONS

Injections are of great value in many situations. This is particularly the case in the treatment of trigger points and tender attachment tissues. They are increasingly used in the treatment of zygoapophyseal joint problems. Caudal epidurals are not only of value in the treatment of lumbar disc lesions, but also in other cases of back pain, because of the number of structures affected by this technique. All these injections are fully described in our companion volume, *An Introduction to Medical Manipulation*[53].

MANIPULATION

This form of therapy is as old as is massage, and works in the same way (i.e. by mechanoceptor stimulation). Thus it now has a scientific backing hitherto lacking, thereby becoming more acceptable and of considerable interest to the medical profession. A practical selection of these techniques is fully described and discussed in our companion volume[53].

References

1. Schultz, A. (1982). Colt Symposium, London
2. Kellgren, J. H. (1939). On the distribution of pain arising from deep somatic structures with charts of segmental pain areas. *Clin. Sci.*, **4**, 35
3. Frykholm, R. (1971). The clinical picture. In Hirsch, C. and Zotterman, Y. (eds.) *Cervical Pain*. p. 5. (Oxford: Pergamon)
4. Cloward, R. B. (1959). Cervical diskography. *Ann. Surg.*, **150**, 1052
5. Holt, E. P. (1964). Fallacy of cervical discography: report of 50 cases in normal subjects. *J. Am. Med. Assoc.*, **188**, 799
6. Klafta, L. A. and Collis, J. S. (1969). The diagnostic inaccuracy of the pain response in cervical discography. *Clev. Clin. Q.*, **36**, 35
7. Kirk, E. J. and Denny-Brown, D. (1970). Functional variations in dermatomes in the macaque monkey following dorsal root lesions. *J. Comp. Neurol.*, **139**, 307
8. Denny-Brown, D., Kirk, E. J. and Yanagisawa, N. (1973). The tract of Lissauer in relation to sensory transmission in the dorsal horn of the spinal cord in the macaque. *J. Comp. Neurol.*, **151**, 175
9. Last, R. J. (1978). *Anatomy, Regional and Applied.* 6th Edn., p. 27. (Edinburgh and London: Churchill Livingstone)
10. Mooney, V. and Robertson, J. (1976). The facet syndrome. *Clin. Orthop. Relat. Res.*, **115**, 149
11. Bourdillon, J. F. (1973). *Spinal Manipulation.* 2nd Edn. (London: Heinemann)
12. Keele, C. A. and Neil, E. (eds.) (1971). *Samson Wright's Applied Physiology.* 12th Edn. (London: Oxford UP)
13. Macnab, I. (1977). *Backache.* (Baltimore: Williams & Wilkins)
14. O'Brien, J. P. (1979). Anterior spinal tenderness in low back pain syndromes. *Spine*, **4**, 85
15. Grieve, G. P. (1981). *Common Vertebral Joint Problems.* (Edinburgh and London: Churchill Livingstone)
16. Froriep, A. (1843). *Ein Betrag zur Pathologie und Therapie des Rheumatismus.* (Weimar)
17. Gowers, W. R. (1904). Lumbago: its lessons and analogues. *Br. Med. J.*, **1**, 117
18. Copeman, W. S. C. and Ackerman, W. L. (1947). Oedema or herniations of fat lobules as a cause of lumbar and gluteal 'fibrositis'. *Arch. Intern. Med.*, **79**, 22
19. Travell, J., Rinzler, S. H. and Hermann, M. (1942). Pain and disability of the shoulder and arm. *J. Am. Med. Assoc.*, **120**, 417
20. Jayson, M. I. V. (ed.) (1980). *The Lumbar Spine and Back Pain.* 2nd Edn. (Tunbridge Wells: Pitman Medical)
21. Mooney, V., Cairns, D. and Robertson, J. (1976). A system for evaluating and treating chronic back disability. *West. J. Med.*, **124**, 370
22. Melzack, R., Stillwell, D. M. and Fox, E. J. (1977). Trigger points and acupuncture points for pain: correlations and implications. *Pain*, **3**, 23
23. Steindler, A. and Luck, J. V. (1938). Differential diagnosis of pain low in the back. *J. Am. Med. Assoc.*, **110**, 106

REFERENCES

24. Simons, D. G. (1975). Muscle pain syndromes: Part I. *Am. J. Phys. Med.*, **54**, 289
25. Maigne, R. (1976). Un signe évocateur et inattendu de céphalée cervicale: la douleur au pince-roulé du sourcil. *Ann. Med. Phys.*, **4**, 416
26. Jayson, M. I. V. (ed.) (1976). *The Lumbar Spine and Back Pain*. (Tunbridge Wells: Pitman Medical)
27. Campbell, D. G. and Parsons, C. M. (1944). Referred head pain and its concomitants. *J. Nerv. Ment. Dis.*, **99**, 544
28. Trevor-Jones, R. (1964). Osteo-arthritis of the paravertebral joints of the second and third cervical vertebrae as a cause of occipital headaches. *S. Afr. Med. J.*, **38**, 392
29. Dutton, C. B. and Riley, L. H. (1969). Cervical migraine: not merely a pain in the neck. *Am. J. Med.*, **47**, 141
30. Magora, F. *et al.* (1974). An electromyographic investigation of the neck muscles in headache. *Electromyogr. Clin. Neurophysiol.*, **14**, 453
31. Maigne, R. (1968). *Douleurs d'origine vertebrale et traitement par manipulations*. (Paris: L'expansion)
32. Friedman, A. P. (1975). Migraine. *Psychiatr. Ann.*, **5**, 29
33. Sheldon, K. W. (1967). Headache patterns and cervical nerve root compression – a 15-year study of hospitalisation for headache. *Headache*, Jan., 180
34. Cope, S. and Ryan, G. M. S. (1959). Cervical and otolith vertigo. *J. Laryngol. Otol.*, **73**, 113
35. Toglia, J. U., Rosenberg, P. E. and Ronis, M. L. (1969). Vestibular and audiological aspects of whiplash injury and head trauma. *J. Foren. Sci.*, **14**, 219
36. Kosoy, J. and Glassman, A. L. (1974). Audiovestibular findings with cervical spine trauma. *Tex. Med.*, **70**, 66
37. Dionne, J. (1974). Neck torsion nystagmus. *Can. J. Otolaryngol.*, **3**, 37
38. Jackson, R. (1967). Headaches associated with disorders of the cervical spine. *Headache*, **6**, 175
39. Roca, P. D. (1972). Ocular manifestations of whiplash injuries. *Ann. Ophthalmol.*, **4**, 63
40. Lieure, J. A. (1953). Paraplégie du aux manoeuvres d'un chiropracteur. *Rev. Rheum.*, **20**, 708
41. Fossgreen, J. (1984). Presentation at *BAMM Symposium*, London
42. Grant, A. P. and Keegan, D. A. J. (1968). Rib pain – a neglected diagnosis. *Ulster Med. J.*, **37**, 162
43. Marinacci, A. A. and Courville, C. B. (1962). Radicular syndromes simulating intra-abdominal surgical conditions. *Am. Surg.*, **28**, 59
44. Ashby, E. C. (1977). Abdominal pain of spinal origin. *Ann. R. Coll. Surg.*, **59**, 242
45. Wall, P. D. and Melzack, R. (1984). *Textbook of Pain*. (London: Churchill Livingstone)
46. Mooney, V. T. (1977). Facet pathology. In Kent, B. (ed.) *Proceedings: Third Seminar: International Federation of Orthopedic and Manipulative Therapists*. (Hayward, CA: IFOMT)
47. King, J. S. (1977). Randomised trial of the Rees and Shealy methods for the treatment of low back pain. In Buerger, A. A. and Tobis, J. S. (eds.) *Approaches to the Validation of Manipulation Therapy*. p. 70. (Springfield: Thomas)
48. Solonen, K. A. (1957). The sacro-iliac joint in the light of anatomical roentgenological and clinical studies. *Acta Orthop. Scand. Suppl.*, 26

REFERENCES

49. Maigne, Gourjon *et al.* (1969). Film.
50. Wyke, B. D. (1980). In Jayson, M. I. V. (ed.) *The Lumbar Spine and Back Pain.* 2nd Edn. (Tunbridge Wells: Pitman Medical)
51. Weinstein, M. A. *et al.* (1975). Computed tomography in diastematomyelia. *Radiology,* 117, 609
52. Junghans, H. (1977). *Nomenclatura Columnae Veretebralis.* (Stuttgart: Hippokrates-Verlag)
53. Paterson, J. K. and Burn, L. (1985). *An Introduction to Medical Manipulation.* (Lancaster: MTP Press)
54. Nachemson, A. L. (1980). In Jayson, M. I. V. (ed.) *The Lumbar Spine and Back Pain.* 2nd Edn. (Tunbridge Wells: Pitman Medical)
55. Cust, G., Pearson, J. C. G. and Mair, A. (1972). The prevalence of low back pain in nurses. *Int. Nurs. Rev.,* 19, 169
56. Huskisson, E. C. (1974). Recent drugs and the rheumatic diseases. *Report on Rheumatic Disease No. 54.* (London: Arthritis and Rheumatism Council)
57. Dick, C. W. (1978). In Scott, J. T. (ed.) *Copeman's Textbook of the Rheumatic Diseases.* 5th Edn. (Edinburgh and London: Churchill Livingstone)
58. Lee, P. *et al.* (1974). Observations on drug prescribing in rheumatoid arthritis. *Br. Med. J.,* 1, 424
59. Rooney, P. J. *et al.* (1975). A short term, double blind controlled trial of prenozone in rheumatoid arthritis. *Curr. Med. Res. Opin.,* 2, 43
60. Basmajian, J. V. and Deluca, C. J. (1985). *Muscles Alive.* (Baltimore: Williams & Wilkins)
61. Jayson, M. (1982). Presentation at *Colt Symposium*
62. Nachemson, A. L. (1976). In Jayson, M. (ed.) *The Lumbar Spine and Back Pain.* (Tunbridge Wells: Pitman Medical)
63. Nathan, H. and Feuerstein, M. (1970). Angulated course of spinal nerve roots. *J. Neurosurg.,* 32, 349
64. Brodal, A. (1965). *The Cranial Nerves – Anatomy and Anatomicoclinical Correlations.* (Oxford: Blackwell Scientific)
65. Brain, Lord and Wilkinson, M. (eds.) (1967). *Cervical Spondylosis.* (London: Heinemann)
66. Wyke, B. D. (1983). Presentation at *7th International Congress of FIMM,* Zürich
67. Andersson, B. J. G., Otengren, R. *et al.* (1974). On myoelectric back muscle activity and lumbar disc pressure in sitting postures. *Scand. J. Rehabil. Med. Suppl.*
68. Farhni, W. H. (1966). *Backache and Primal Posture.* (Vancouver: Musqueam Publishers)
69. McKenzie, R. A. (1977). Prophylaxis in recurrent low back pain. In *Proceedings: International Federation of Manual Medicine Congress, Copenhagen*
70. Nachemson, A. (1976). The lumbar spine; an orthopaedic challenge. *Spine,* 1, 59
71. Weinstein, P. R., Ehni, G. and Wilson, C. B. (1977). *Lumbar Spondylosis: Diagnosis, Management and Surgical Treatment.* (Chicago and London: Year Book Medical)
72. Hutton, W. C. and Adams, M. A. (1980). The forces acting on the neural arch and their relevance to low back pain. In *Conference Proceedings: Engineering Aspects of the Spine.* p. 49. (London: Mechanical Engineering Publications)
73. Wood, P. H. N. (1976). The epidemiology of back pain. In Jayson, M. (ed.) *The Lumbar Spine and Back Pain.* p. 13. (Tunbridge Wells: Pitman Medical)
74. Troup, J. D. G. (1979). Biomechanics of the vertebral column. *Physiotheraphy,* 65, 238

123

REFERENCES

75. Kendall *et al.* (1971). Cited in ref. 60
76. Edwards and Hyde (1977). Cited in ref. 60
77. Sternbach, R. A. (1974). *Pain Patients. Traits and Treatment.* (New York: Academic Press)
78. Woodforde, J. M. and Merskey, H. (1972). Personality traits of patients with chronic pain. *J. Psychosom. Res.,* **16,** 167–72
79. Engel, G. L. 'Psychogenic' pain and the pain-prone patient. *Am. J. Med.,* **26,** 899–918
80. Hilton, R. C. (1980). In Jayson, M. (ed.) *The Lumbar Spine and Back Pain.* 2nd Edn. (Tunbridge Wells: Pitman Medical)
81. Moll, J. and Wright, V. (1980). In Jayson, M. (ed.) *The Lumbar Spine and Back Pain.* 2nd Edn. (Tunbridge Wells: Pitman Medical)
82. Dvorak, J., Dvorak, V. and Schneider, W. (1984). *Manual Medicine 1984.* (Berlin: Springer Verlag)

Index

legs
  apparent differences in length 91–2
  straight leg raising 57–8
lifting 119
ligamentous pain 20
limb muscles, mechanoceptive reflex effects
  8, 9
lordosis 47, 119
low back pain
  and posture 119
  classification 17
  defined 17
  primary backache 17–22
  psychosomatic backache 27–8
  referred backache 14, 25–7
  secondary backache 22–5
  thoracic source 31
lumbar region
  data recording 108–11
  examination 47–58
  global movements 48–51
  paravertebral muscle tone test 83
  pressure tests 84–6
  skin drag test 81
  skin pinching test 82–3
  zygoapophyseal tenderness test 86
lumbar spine
  examination 59
  indications for surgery 62–3
  referred pain 31

manipulation 5, 120
  reaction of mechanoceptors 2
massage 4, 116
  stimulation of mechanoceptors 120
mechanoceptors 2
  behaviour at rest or when moved 2
  experimental reactions to stimuli 7–9
  pain inhibition 5
  path of afferent fibres 3, 4
  rates of adaptation 2
  reaction to manipulation 2
  reaction to traction 2
  stimulation by massage 120
  therapeutic stimulation of afferent
    fibres 4–5
migraine, and cervical spine involvement 29
mobility testing 66, 93
muscle fatigue
  in primary backache 19
  relief of 19
muscle spasm
  in cervical region 33
  in lumbar region 47
  in primary backache 18
  in thoracic region 46

muscles
  assessing power reduction 41–5, 47
  in lumbar region 52–4
  compensatory activity 12
  examination 93
  function and interaction 11
  function assessment methods 11
  paravertebral muscle tone test 67, 72,
    77, 83
  testing 66–7
myelopathy
  cervical 62
  thoracic 62

neck pain 62
nerve endings
  classification 2
  see also mechanoceptors; nociceptors
nerve root damage, and tendon reflexes
  39–41
nociceptors
  experimental reactions to stimuli 7–9
  irritation 3
  in primary backache 17, 18
  path of afferent fibres 3, 4, 5

osteomalacia 21
osteoporosis 21

pain
  basic neurology 1–6
  in primary backache 17
  inhibition by mechanoceptive input 5
  perception 3–4, 5
palpation, deep 67, 73
  lumbar region 84
  pelvis 89
  thoracic region 77
paravertebral muscle tone test 67
  cervical region 72
  lumbar region 83
  thoracic region 77
pelvic ligament tests 59–61
pelvic region
  data recording 112–13
  examination 58–61
  tests 87–90
pelvic tilt 47
peritoneal disorders, and referred backache
  25
personality testing 27
polymyalgia rheumatica 63
posture
  and primary back pain 20
  cervical 33–5
  lumbar 47